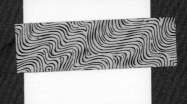

Surgical Management of
Pelvic Organ Prolapse

FEMALE PELVIC SURGERY VIDEO ATLAS SERIES
Series Editor:

Mickey Karram, MD
Director of Urogynecology
The Christ Hospital
Clinical Professor of Obstetrics and Gynecology and Urology
University of Cincinnati
Cincinnati, Ohio

Other Volumes in the Female Pelvic Surgery Video Atlas Series

FEMALE PELVIC SURGERY VIDEO ATLAS SERIES
Mickey Karram, Series Editor

Surgical Management of Pelvic Organ Prolapse

Mickey Karram, MD
Director of Urogynecology
The Christ Hospital
Clinical Professor of Obstetrics and Gynecology and Urology
University of Cincinnati
Cincinnati, Ohio

Christopher F. Maher, MD
Wesley and Royal Brisbane Urogynaecology Unit
Brisbane, Queensland
Australia

Illustrated by **Joe Chovan, Milford, Ohio**

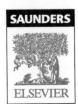

SAUNDERS

ELSEVIER

1600 John F. Kennedy Blvd.
Ste 1800
Philadelphia, PA 19103-2899

SURGICAL MANAGEMENT OF PELVIC ORGAN PROLAPSE ISBN: 978-1-4160-6266-0

Library of Congress Cataloging-in-Publication Data
Karram, Mickey M.
 Surgical management of pelvic organ prolapse / Mickey Karram, Christopher F. Maher.—1st ed.
   p. ; cm.—(Female pelvic surgery video atlas series)
 Includes bibliographical references and index.
 ISBN 978-1-4160-6266-0 (hardback)
 I. Maher, Christopher F. II. Title. III. Series: Female pelvic surgery video atlas series.
 [DNLM: 1. Pelvic Organ Prolapse—surgery. 2. Genital Diseases, Female—surgery. WP 468]
 618.1'44059—dc23

                                                    2012025961

Senior Content Strategist: Stefanie Jewell-Thomas
Senior Content Development Specialist: Arlene Chappelle
Publishing Services Manager: Patricia Tannian
Project Manager: Anita Somaroutu
Design Direction: Louis Forgione

To the women in my life; my wife, Mona, for her unyielding support, love, and dedication to our family unit; and to my three daughters, Tamara, Lena, and Summer, for the joy they give me on a daily basis.

—Mickey Karram

To my parents, Christopher and Clare Maher, for instilling in me from a young age the importance of perseverance and dedication in attaining goals.
To my lovely wife, Dympna, for her enduring love and support and for allowing me the freedom to strive for these goals.
To my children, Hannah, Malachy, Declan, and Clare, for the great joy of being their father and for teaching me the importance of always re-evaluating goals.
Finally, to all my fellows and students, for continually reactivating and refreshing my desire to strive for excellence in the management of female pelvic floor dysfunction.

—Christopher F. Maher

Contributors

Mickey Karram, MD
Director of Urogynecology, The Christ Hospital, Clinical Professor of Obstetrics and Gynecology, University of Cincinnati, Cincinnati, Ohio
2: Surgical Anatomy of the Pelvis and the Anatomy of Pelvic Support; 3: Preoperative Evaluation and Staging of Patients with Pelvic Organ Prolapse; 4: Techniques for Vaginal Hysterectomy and Vaginal Trachelectomy in Patients with Pelvic Organ Prolapse; 5: Surgical Procedures to Suspend a Prolapsed Uterus; 7: Surgical Management of Apical Vaginal Prolapse; 8: Surgical Management of Anterior Vaginal Wall Prolapse; 9: Surgical Correction of Posterior Pelvic Floor Defects; 10: Obliterative Procedures for Pelvic Organ Prolapse; 11: Surgery for Pelvic Organ Prolapse: Avoiding and Managing Complications

Christopher F. Maher, MD
Wesley and Royal Brisbane Urogynaecology Unit, Brisbane, Queensland, Australia
1: Epidemiology, Risk Factors, and Social Impact of Pelvic Organ Prolapse; 5: Surgical Procedures to Suspend a Prolapsed Uterus; 7: Surgical Management of Apical Vaginal Wall Prolapse; 8: Surgical Management of Anterior Vaginal Wall Prolapse; 11: Surgery for Pelvic Organ Prolapse: Avoiding and Managing Complications

Janelle Evans, MD
Urogynecology Fellow, The Christ Hospital, Cincinnati, Ohio
10: Obliterative Procedures for Pelvic Organ Prolapse

Catherine A. Matthews, MD
Division of Urogynecology and Reconstructive Pelvic Surgery, University of North Carolina, Chapel Hill, North Carolina
6: Robot-Assisted Laparoscopic Colposacropexy and Cervicosacropexy

Corina Schmid, MD
Urogynaecology Fellow, RBWH Department for Urogynaecology, Herston, Queensland, Australia
1: Epidemiology, Risk Factors, and Social Impact of Pelvic Organ Prolapse

Video Contributors

Chi Chiung Grace Chen, MD
Assistant Professor, Department of Obstetrics and Gynecology, Johns Hopkins Bayview Medical Center, Baltimore, Maryland
Video: *Morcellation Techniques in Patients with an Unsuspected Enlarged Uterus*

Gouri D. Diwadkar, MD
Fellow, Female Pelvic Medicine and Reconstructive Surgery, Department of Obstetrics and Gynecology; Obstetrics, Gynecology, and Women's Health Institute, Cleveland Clinic, Cleveland, Ohio
Video: *Morcellation Techniques in Patients with an Unsuspected Enlarged Uterus*

Anna C. Frick, MD
Fellow, Female Pelvic Medicine and Reconstructive Surgery, Center for Urogynecology and Reconstructive Pelvic Surgery, Obstetrics, Gynecology, and Women's Health Institute, Cleveland Clinic, Cleveland, Ohio
Video: *Electrosurgical Device-Assisted Vaginal Hysterectomy*

Roger Goldberg, MD, MPH
Clinical Associate Professor, University of Chicago Pritzker School of Medicine, NorthShore University HealthSystem, Division of Urogynecology, Evanston, Illinois
Video: *Uphold Uterine Suspension*

Paul Moran, BMedSci, BM, BS
Consultant Gynaecologist, Worcestershire Royal Hospital, Worcester, United Kingdom
Video: *Anterior Repair with Midline Fascial Plication*

Tristi W. Muir, MD
Associate Professor, Department of Obstetrics and Gynecology, Director, Urogynecology, University of Texas Medical Branch, Galveston, Texas
Video: *Technique for Vaginal Oophorectomy*

Marie Fidela R. Paraiso, MD
Section Head, Center of Urogynecology and Reconstructive Pelvic Surgery, Obstetrics, Gynecology, and Women's Health Institute, Cleveland Clinic, Cleveland, Ohio
Video: *Morcellation Techniques in Patients with an Unsuspected Enlarged Uterus*

Bob Shull, MD
Department of Obstetrics and Gynecology, Texas A&M University System Health Science Center, Pelvic Reconstructive Surgery, Scott & White Healthcare, Temple Clinic, Temple, Texas
Video: *Postoperative Management of Ureteral Obstruction after Vaginal Prolapse Repair*

Mark D. Walters, MD
Professor and Vice Chair of Gynecology, Department of Obstetrics and Gynecology, Obstetrics, Gynecology, and Women's Health Institute, Cleveland Clinic, Cleveland, Ohio
Video: *Morcellation Techniques in Patients with an Unsuspected Enlarged Uterus; Technique for Vaginal Oophorectomy; Electrosurgical Device-Assisted Vaginal Hysterectomy*

Preface

Vaginal reconstructive surgery is concerned with the return of abnormal organ relationships to a usual or normal state. There is no one site or degree of damage that must be repaired or restored; there are many and they occur in various combinations at various times of life from different etiologic factors, in varying degrees and with varying degrees of symptoms and disability."

Nichols and Randall, 1989

This statement, made over 20 years ago, eloquently relays the complexities involved in surgically managing patients with pelvic organ prolapse. One in 10 women in the United States will undergo a prolapse repair in their lifetime, and up to 50% of parous women develop prolapse with symptoms. With the aging female being the largest growing segment of the population, these numbers will only increase over time.

At present, there are significant differences in opinion among pelvic surgeons on how best to surgically correct symptomatic pelvic organ prolapse. While the ultimate goal of any reconstructive pelvic surgery is to restore anatomy, restore or maintain bladder and bowel function, and restore or maintain sexual function (if desired), obtaining and eventually objectifying these outcomes have proven to be extremely challenging endeavors.

This book is part of the eight-book series, "Female Pelvic Surgery Video Atlas Series." This text, in line with the others in the series, is designed to be a how-to guide for the various procedures and techniques used to correct pelvic organ prolapse. Although all procedures cannot be described in great detail, the authors have chosen the procedures that have worked well in their hands as well as procedures that have been shown to be successful in the literature. The text is accompanied by numerous original illustrations by renowned medical illustrator Joe Chovan as well as more than 70 videos demonstrating the various techniques discussed and illustrated in the text.

We have tried to create a text that is comprehensive and objective yet clinically oriented by presenting the various techniques in a clinical case format that highlights the technical aspects of the procedure as well as preoperative preparation and postoperative management. We have tried to address controversial topics, such as route of surgery and mesh augmentation, in an objective, unbiased fashion.

The book begins with a review of epidemiology, risk factors, and social impact of pelvic organ prolapse. Chapter 2 discusses surgical anatomy of pelvic organ support. This chapter is accompanied by numerous video clips of cadaveric dissections as well as live surgical demonstrations to facilitate a three-dimensional anatomic understanding of the anatomy of pelvic support. Chapter 3 reviews the methods to use in the preoperative assessment of patients with pelvic organ prolapse as well as commonly utilized staging techniques for documenting the severity of prolapse. Chapter 4 discusses and demonstrates techniques for simple and difficult vaginal hysterectomy and trachelectomy. Chapter 5 reviews hysteropexy with a detailed discussion and demonstration of laparoscopic and vaginal techniques. Chapter 6 discusses the use of robotic-assisted laparoscopic colposacropexy and cervicosacropexy. Chapters 7 through 9 review the surgical management of anterior, apical, and posterior vaginal wall prolapse. These chapters include detailed discussions on laparoscopic and abdominal approaches to mesh augmentation, vaginal approaches to mesh augmentation, and native tissue vaginal suture repairs. Chapter 10 reviews obliterative procedures with detailed discussions on the LeFort partial colpocleisis and complete colpectomy and colpocleisis. Chapter 11 presents a series of 15 cases related to various complications that can occur with prolapse procedures. All the cases are accompanied by a surgical video clip to illustrate fully how best to avoid and manage the specific complication.

We hope this text and unique method of presenting information will be well received by reconstructive surgeons, whether they are residents or fellows or are more seasoned gynecologic or urogynecologic surgeons. The ultimate hope is to improve the skill level of all surgeons managing these common disorders.

Mickey Karram
Christopher F. Maher

Contents

Epidemiology, Risk Factors, and Social Impact of Pelvic Organ Prolapse

Corina Schmid MD and Christopher F. Maher MD

Introduction

Pelvic organ prolapse (POP) is a common problem affecting up to 50% of parous women; 6.3% of women will undergo a surgical correction for POP by 80 years of age. Prolapse surgery is an increasingly important part of gynecologic practice as a result of an aging population and the decreasing rate of hysterectomies. Prolapse surgery is already performed twice as frequently as continence surgery, and the surgical and admission times are at least three times greater than continence surgery. Considering the increasing time and resources devoted to POP, surprisingly little is known regarding the incidence, prevalence, risk factors, and progression rates of this condition.

POP is defined by the International Continence Society (ICS) as the descent of one or more of the following structures: the anterior or posterior vaginal wall, the apex of the vagina, or the vault. Loss of the vaginal support is observed in 43% to 76% of patients during routine gynecologic care and in up to 3% to 6% with a descent beyond the hymen. (Swift et al, 2005; Samuelsson et al, 1999)

Prevalence and Incidence of Pelvic Organ Prolapse

Epidemiologic studies of the natural history, incidence, and prevalence of POP are currently lacking. It is widely accepted that 50% of women will develop prolapse, but only 10% to 20% of those will seek evaluation for their condition. (Phillips et al, 2006) In the current literature, the overall prevalence of POP shows significant variation, depending on the definition used, ranging from 3% to 50% (Table 1-1). When POP is defined and graded on symptoms, the prevalence is 3% to 6%, as compared with 41% to 50% when based on examination, indicating that the majority of women with prolapse are asymptomatic. (Phillips et al, 2006; Samuelsson et al, 1999; Nygaard et al, 2008; Swift, Tate, Nicholas, 2003) On examination, anterior compartment prolapse is the most frequently reported site of prolapse, is detected twice as often as posterior compartment defects, and three times more often than apical prolapse. (Hendrix et al, 2002; Handa et al, 2004) After hysterectomy, 6% to 12% of women will develop vault prolapse (Marchionni et al, 1999; Aigmueller et al, 2010), and in two thirds of these cases, multiple compartment prolapse is present. (Morley, DeLancey, 1988)

Little knowledge of the natural history of POP is available. The reported incidence for cystocele is approximately 9 per 100 women-years, 6 per 100 women-years for rectocele, and 1.5 per 100 women-years for uterine prolapse. (Handa et al, 2004) Bradley et al, report the 1-year incidence of POP at 26% and the 3-year incidence at 40% with regression rates of 21% and 19%, respectively. In general, older parous women are more likely to develop new or progressive POP than to show regression. Of the women over 65 years of age, 10% have had prolapse progression of more than 2 cm, whereas only 2.7% of women younger than 65 years had a regression by the same amount. (Bradley et al, 2007)

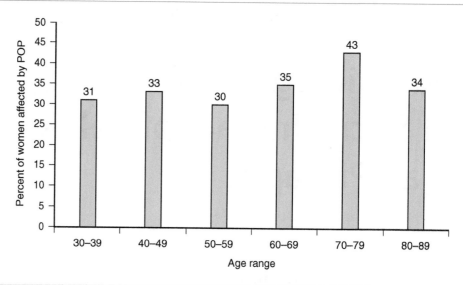

Figure 1-1 Distribution of pelvic organ prolapse (POP) among women seeking care in the United States (2000).

Table 1-1 Prevalence and Incidence

Study	Definition	Prevalence	Incidence	Country
Rortveit, 2007	Symptom based	5.7%		U.S.
Nygaard, 2008	Symptom based	2.9%		U.S.
Hendrix, 2002	WHI Study, Examination	Any prolapse: 41.1% Cystocele: 34.3% Rectocele: 18.6% Uterine: 14.2%		U.S.
Swift, 2003	Examination	Stage 0: 6.4% Stage 1: 43.3% Stage 2: 47.7% Stage 3: 2.6%		U.S.
Handa, 2004	WHI Study, Examination	Cystocele: 24.6% Rectocele: 12.9% Uterine: 3.8%	Cystocele: 9.3/100 Rectocele: 5.7/100 Uterine: 1.5/100	U.S.
Nygaard, 2004	Examination	Stage 0: 2.3% Stage 1: 33% Stage 2: 63% Stage 3: 1.9%		U.S.
Bradley, 2007	Examination	23.5%-49.9%	26%/1 year 40%/3 year	US
Marchionni, 1999	Examination	Vault-prolapse: 12%		Italy
Aigmueller, 2010	Examination	Vault-prolapse: 6%-8%		Austria

Adapted from Sung and Hampton 2009.

In a large demographic study, Luber and associates (2001) have shown that the peak incidence of symptoms attributed to prolapse is between the ages of 70 and 79 years, whereas POP symptoms are still relatively common in women of younger age (Figure 1-1).

Demographic changes with an aging population have significant implications for the future planning of women's health services. Wu and colleagues (2009) have predicted that by 2050 the number of women suffering from symptomatic POP in the United States will increase at minimum by 46% (from 3.3 to 4.9 million women) and, in a "worst-case scenario," up to 200% or 9.2 million women with POP.

Incidence and Prevalence of Prolapse Surgery

Both incidence and prevalence for prolapse surgery increase with age. Women older than 80 years of age are currently the fastest growing segment of the population. The

Figure 1-2 Surgical treatment for pelvic organ prolapse (POP) per 10,000 women (2003) and obesity.

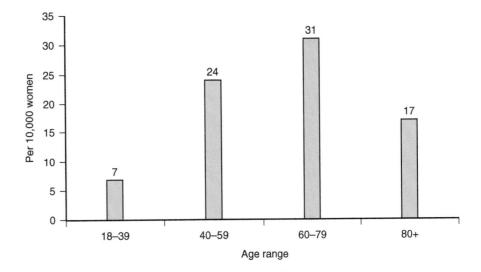

estimated lifetime risk of an American woman undergoing at least one surgical intervention by the age of 80 years is 6.3% with 30% requiring subsequent surgeries. (Olsen et al, 1997) However, a more recent prospective study showed a significantly lower subsequent surgical rate of only 13%, which may be explained by improved surgical procedures. (Clark et al, 2003) The longevity or durability of POP surgery is an important variable for planning and thus requires ongoing evaluation.

The annual incidence for POP surgery is reported to be between 1.5 (Boyles, 2003) and 1.8 (Shah et al, 2007) cases per 1000 women-years with the incidence peaking in women between the ages of 60 and 69 years. Shah and associates (2007) also demonstrated a peak incidence in 70-year-old women. However, Luber and colleagues (2001) reported surprisingly high numbers of younger women who were also undergoing surgical treatments with a similarity in the prolapse symptoms (Figure 1-2). A more recent study by Smith and associates (2010) reported a lifetime risk of undergoing prolapse surgery as high as 19% in Western Australia. This figure is three times higher than the 6.3% lifetime risk for POP surgery reported by Olsen and others (1997) and requires further evaluation of local factors, as well as other definitions that may have contributed.

In the United States, POP is thought to be the leading cause for more than 300,000 surgical procedures per year (22.7 per 10,000 women) with 25% undergoing subsequent surgical procedures at a total annual cost of more than 1 billion dollars. (Brown et al, 2002; Boyles, Weber, Meyn, 2003; Silva et al, 2006; Shah et al, 2007) Also of note is a study during a 9-year period (1996 to 2005) that reported an increase of 40% of the ambulatory costs related to pelvic floor disorders; if these figures are extrapolated to POP surgery costs, the total annual cost would be over 1.4 billion dollars.

The incidence of prolapse requiring surgical correction after a hysterectomy is 3.6 per 1000 women-years, according to a large cohort study conducted by Mant and colleagues (1997) in the United Kingdom. The cumulative risk rises to 5% 15 years after hysterectomy.

Etiologic Features and Risk Factors of Pelvic Organ Prolapse

The etiologic features of POP are still poorly understood and multifactorial, attributable to a combination of risk factors and varying from patient to patient. (Schaffer, 2005) A reduction of the stability of the pelvic floor muscles and connective tissue through tearing, trauma, and chronically raised intraabdominal pressure are likely to be the key mechanisms involved in the development of POP (Table 1-2).

Vaginal birth, advancing age, and an increased body mass index (BMI) or obesity are known to be the most consistent risk factors of developing uterogenital prolapse;

Table 1-2 Risk Factors for the Development of Pelvic Organ Prolapse

Factors	Impact on the Development Pelvic Organ Prolapse
Vaginal delivery, parity	RR two children: 8.4* RR four children: 10.9* 10%-20% every additional child
Strong family history	Mother: OR 3.2 (95% CI 1.1-7.6) Sister: OR 2.4 (95% CI 1.0-5.6)
Advancing age	60-69 years of age: OR 1.2 (95% CI 1.0-1.3) 70-79 years of age: OR 1.4 (95% CI 1.2-1.6)
Connective tissue disorder	Marfan syndrome: 33% Ehlers-Danlos syndrome: 75% Hernias: 31%
Overweight Obesity Chronic increase of intraabdominal pressure	2.51 (95% CI 1.18-5.35) 2.56 (95% CI 1.23-5.33) Physical work: OR 2.0 (95% CI 1.1-3.6)
Previous gynecologic surgery	Posthysterectomy POP: 6%-12% Postcolposuspension: 30% risk for rectocele or apex descent
Racial differences	Caucasian: 5.35 (95% CI 1.89-15.12) for POP Hispanics: 4.89 (95% CI 1.64-14.58) for POP

*As compared to nulliparous women.
CI, Confidence interval; OR, odds ratio; POP, pelvic organ prolapse; RR, relative risk.

however, numerous other factors contribute to this condition. The incidence of POP is largely correlated to **vaginal birth**, which is well documented in epidemiologic and cohort studies. (Nygaard et al, 2008; Rortveit et al, 2007) Vaginal delivery leads to tearing, stretching, and the dislocation of the pelvic muscles and nerves. In the Oxford Family Planning Study, increasing vaginal parity was the most relevant and strongest risk factor for POP in women younger than 60 years of age. Women who had two or four children delivered vaginally had a relative risk (RR) of developing a POP of 8.4 and 10.9, respectively, as compared with nulliparous women. Hendrix and associates (2002) showed similar findings, reporting that each additional childbirth increases the risk of developing POP by 10% to 20%. Forceps delivery, high infant birth weight, prolonged second stage, and young age (under 25 years old) at the first pregnancy are considered additional obstetric risk factors for POP but less than vaginal childbirth and parity. (Swift, Tate, Nicholas, 2003; Moalli et al, 2003)

Elective Cesarean section reduces the incidence of POP. Women who have undergone vaginal delivery have a higher risk of developing prolapse symptoms as compared to those who had elective cesarian section (RR 1.82 95% CI 1.04 to 3.19). These data estimate that for every seven women with elective cesarean section, one woman would be prevented from developing a pelvic organ disorder. (Lukacz et al, 2006) With the steadily increasing number of elective cesarean sections, and thus the decreasing numbers of vaginal deliveries, a reduction in the incidence of POP may be achieved in the future.

The question of whether pregnancy, itself, is to be considered a risk factor is controversially discussed in the literature. Small studies show trends toward a worsening prolapse rate after pregnancy—distinct from the mode of delivery—compared with nonpregnant control groups. However, prolapse can also be seen in nulliparous women; therefore other factors must be involved in the development of prolapse, which supports the multifactorial model of the genesis of POP.

Advancing age is strongly associated with POP. Both prevalence and the incidence significantly increase with age. Progressing denervation of the pelvic floor muscles with age may contribute to POP. (Wall, 1993) The relative prevalence of POP rises approximately 40% with every decade of life. (Swift et al, 2005) The Women's Health Initiative (WHI) stated that the risk for developing POP in women between ages 60 and 69 years and between ages 70 and 79 years (odds ratio [OR] 1.2; 95% CI 1.0 to 1.3 and OR 1.4; 95% CI 1.2 to 1.6 respectively) is higher than women aged 50 to 59 years of age.

Obesity and conditions of chronically increased intraabdominal pressure, such as constipation, asthma, chronic obstructive pulmonary disease (COPD), and regular weightlifting, place excessive strain on the pelvic floor, supporting muscles, connective tissues, and pudendal nerves. (Swift, Tate, Nicholas, 2003; Spence-Jones et al, 1994) As a result, women who are overweight or obese are at high risk of developing POP with an OR of 2.51 (95% CI 1.18 to 5.35) and 2.56 (95% CI 1.23 to 5.35), respectively. Similarly, overweight women (BMI greater than 26 kg/m^2) are more than 1.5 to 5.9 times more likely to undergo prolapse surgery than those with normal BMI. (Moalli et al, 2003; Swift, Tate, Nicholas, 2003; Hendrix et al, 2002) The obesity epidemic in developed countries will further challenge POP surgeons in the future.

Other conditions with chronically increased intraabdominal pressure, such as chronic constipation or straining to defecate as a young adult, are highly associated with the development of prolapse when compared with women with normal bowel function (61% versus 4%). Many women who have physically demanding jobs such as nurses, cleaners, or caregivers are twice as likely to develop POP, as compared with sedentary women. (Miedel et al, 2009) These women have a high chance of undergoing a surgical procedure for POP.

The association between a strong family history and prolapse, increased prevalence of hernias in patients with POP, racial differences in the prevalence of prolapse, and the increased prevalence in women with a connective tissue disorder (e.g., Marfan syndrome) make it very likely that **genetic factors** play an important role in the etiologic development of POP.

Quantitative and qualitative differences in collagen are likely to contribute to POP. Some histopathologic studies have showed that women with POP have proportionally more type III collagen than other subtypes. (Moalli et al, 2005) Jackson and associates (1996) found in premenopausal women with POP a reduction of total collagen and secondary increased collagenolytic activity in samples of vaginal tissue, as compared with those without prolapse. Differences in collagen structure may possibly account for the strong familial links to prolapse development. Women with a first-degree family history for this condition have a much higher risk for developing POP with a mother OR 3.2 (95% CI 1.1 to 7.6) or a sister OR 2.4 (95% CL 1.0 to 5.6) reporting prolapse. (Brown et al, 2002; Chiaffarino et al, 1999)

POP and **hernias** share similar pathophysiologic features. Patients with hernias show a decreased collagen synthesis metabolism, a protease-antiprotease imbalance with increased matrix metalloproteinases activity, and a reduced collagen type I/III ratio. Segev and colleagues (2009) demonstrated that women with POP have a significantly higher total prevalence of hernias (31.6% versus 5%, $p = 0.0002$), compared with women with mild or no prolapse.

In terms of **racial** or **ethnical differences**, studies have shown that African-American women have a lower prevalence of POP than Caucasian-American women (Luber, Boero, Choe, 2001; Shah et al, 2007; Whitcombe et al, 2009) with a prevalence ratio of 5.35 (95% CI 1.89 to 15.12) and 4.89 (95% CI 1.64 to 14.58) for symptomatic prolapse in Caucasian and Latina women, respectively. This prevalence may be the result of a smaller pelvic outlet, compared with women from European descent.

Connective tissue disorders, such as Ehlers-Danlos syndrome and Marfan syndrome with an impaired collagen and elastin synthesis and metabolism, have a higher rate of POP. In a small cohort study, 33% of women with Marfan syndrome and 75% with Ehlers-Danlos syndrome developed POP. These findings underline the hypothesis that connective tissue disorders play an important role in the cause of POP. (Carley, Schaffer, 2000)

Prior pelvic surgery may also be a risk factor for subsequential POP surgery, depending on the indications. Approximately 7% of women who have undergone a **previous hysterectomy** are considered at risk for subsequential POP. (Moalli et al, 2003; Mant, Painter, Vessey, 1997) The risk of developing recurrent or nontreated compartmental prolapse is 5.5 times higher in women whose primary indication for hysterectomy was prolapse. Similarly, Dällenbach and others (2007) showed that the risk of subsequential prolapse surgery was 4.7 times higher in women whose initial hysterectomy was for prolapse and 8.0 times higher if preoperative prolapse stage II or more was present.

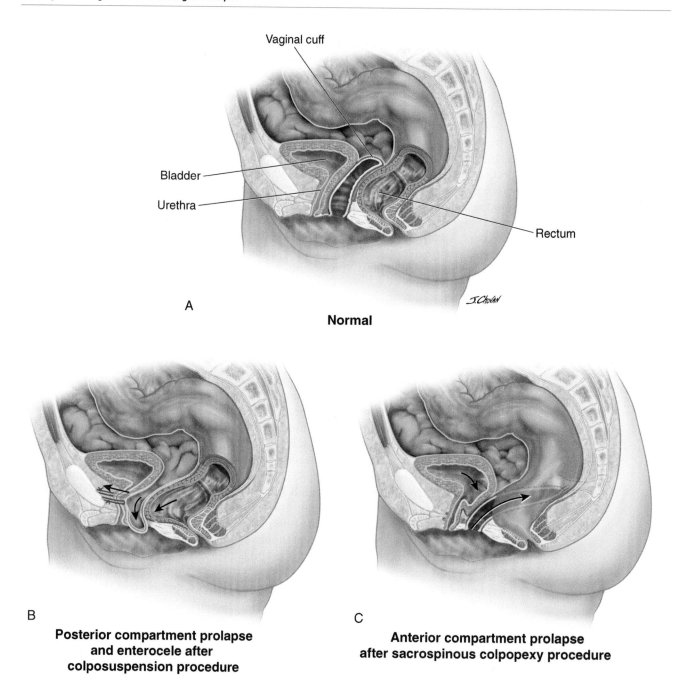

Figure 1-3 A, Normal vaginal topography. **B,** Elevated vaginal mucosa after colposuspension predisposes to iatrogenic posterior compartmental prolapse. **C,** Retroverted vaginal apex after sacrospinous colpopexy predisposes to iatrogenic anterior compartmental prolapse.

(From Nitti VW: Vaginal surgery for the urologist. In Karram M, editor: Female pelvic surgery video atlas series, Philadelphia, 2012, Elsevier.)

Prior pelvic surgery or iatrogenic prolapse is well reported with anterior compartmental prolapse observed in up to one third of women after sacrospinous colpopexy; in addition, posterior compartmental defects increased by one third in those who undergo colposuspension as compared to suburethral tape continence surgery (Figure 1-3). (Ward, Hilton, UK and Ireland TVT Trial Group, 2008) More recently, a single study found that *de novo* POP greater than the Pelvic Organ Prolapse Quantification (POPQ) system stage II occurred in 46% after an isolated anterior vaginal mesh repair and 25% after an isolated posterior vaginal mesh repair. These prevalence rates are of great concern, and further evaluation of the use of mesh in prolapse surgery is urgently indicated. (Withagen, Vierhout, Milani, 2010)

Social Impact of Pelvic Organ Prolapse

As the population of older women constantly increases, the national burden in terms of economic resources, health costs, and productivity caused by decreased quality of life will be substantial. POP can affect a patient's quality of life in many ways. However, no clear correlation exists between the extent of the prolapse and the symptoms caused; however, evidence suggests that women with the leading edge of the prolapse beyond the hymenal remnants have increased symptoms. (Swift, Tate, Nicholas, 2003) Some women are more handicapped and bothered by a mild prolapse than patients with a long-lasting history of an extensive prolapse. The significant variation in the impact that POP has on women mandates that the clinician completes a standardized history, preferably with patient-completed validated questionnaires and careful examination to ensure that any prolapse is actually contributing to the symptom complex.

Numerous validated questionnaires assess the impact of POP on the different aspects of the quality of life. The most commonly used assessment tools are the short form of the Pelvic Floor Distress Inventory (PFDI-20) and the Pelvic Floor Impact Questionnaire (PFIQ-7); both are reliable, comprehensive, and valid condition-specific tools that assess the quality of life in patients with pelvic floor disorders including POP, urinary incontinence, and fecal incontinence. (Barber, Walters, Bump, 2005)

Women suffering from symptomatic prolapse may reduce activities; for example, walking or going to the gym may be avoided because of the dragging of the vagina or cycling may be reduced because of the pain. Older women who are caregivers to loved ones and required to perform heavy lifting are at danger of developing POP. Women deferring these activities to minimize the impact of prolapse are impairing their quality of life, and these decisions have enormous social and economic effects. Although no direct evidence directly links POP to depression, evidence suggests that women have clinically significant improvement in vitality, mental health, social functioning, and role-emotion after prolapse surgery. (Barber et al, 2007)

Apart from the dragging sensation and the feeling of a full vagina, some women with POP are suffering from urinary or bowel symptoms or both, the most common being obstructive voiding dysfunction, incomplete bladder emptying with recurrent urinary tract infections, and overactive bladder (OAB). Some women also complain of hesitancy and a weak or prolonged urinary stream. These symptoms result in women sexually isolating themselves and refusing to ever go for a walk without knowing the location of the toilets.

Women with predominantly posterior compartmental prolapse may seek medical help because of difficulties with impaired defecation where digital manipulation of the vagina or the anus is required to complete defecation. The impact that the surgical correction of POP will have on both bladder and bowel functions, as well as sexual function, is fully discussed in the following chapters.

Sexual dysfunction is common in patients with POP, and women with a large prolapse are often reluctant to have sexual intercourse. Until recently, little data in the literature concerning the influence of prolapse surgery on sexual function have been available; however, some evidence points toward a positive effect. (Handa et al, 2007)

The Pelvic Organ Prolapse/Urinary Incontinence Sexual Questionnaire (PISQ-31) is a validated and reliable questionnaire that assesses sexual dysfunction in patients with POP or urinary incontinence. (Rogers et al, 2001) It contains 31 questions divided into three domains. A short version containing 12 questions (PISQ-12) has been developed that predicts PISQ-31 scores. (Rogers et al, 2003) Women with POP are more likely to be affected by sexual dysfunction than women with urinary incontinence. (Barber et al, 2002)

In conclusion, the impact that POP has on pelvic floor symptoms shows significant variation, and the clinician needs to inform women which symptoms and problems are attributable to the POP and what impact a surgical correction of POP will have on pelvic floor symptoms.

Suggested Readings

Aigmueller T, Dungl A, Hinterholzer S, et al: An estimation of the frequency of surgery for posthysterectomy vault prolapsed, *Int Urogynecol J* 21:299–302, 2010.

Barber MD, Visco AG, Wyman JF, et al: Sexual function in women with urinary incontinence and pelvic organ prolapse, *Obstet Gynecol* 99(2):281–289, 2002.

Barber MD, Walters MD, Bump RC: Short forms of two condition-specific quality-of-life questionnaires for women with pelvic floor disorders (PFDI-20 and PFIQ-7), *Am J Obstet Gynecol* 193:103–113, 2005.

Barber MD, Amundsen CL, Paraiso MF, et al: Quality of life after surgery for genital prolapse in elderly women: obliterative and reconstructive surgery, *Int Urogynecol J Pelvic Floor Dysfunct* 18(7):799–806, 2007.

Boyles SH, Weber AM, Meyn L: Procedures for pelvic organ prolapse in the United States, 1979-1997, *Am J Obstet Gynecol* 188:108–115, 2003.

Boyles SH, Edwards SR: Repair of the anterior vaginal compartment, *Clin Obstet Gynecol* 48(3):682–690, 2005.

Bradley CS, Zimmerman MB, Qi Y, et al: Natural history of pelvic organ prolapse in postmenopausal women, *Obstet Gynecol* 109:848–854, 2007.

Brown JS, Waetjen LE, Subak LL, et al: Pelvic organ prolapse surgery in the United States, 1997, *Am J Obstet Gynecol* 186:712–716, 2002.

Bump RC, Mattiasson A, Bø K, et al: The standardization of terminology of female pelvic organ prolapse and pelvic floor dysfunction, *Am J Obstet Gynecol* 175:10–17, 1996.

Carley ME, Schaffer J: Urinary incontinence and pelvic organ prolapse in women with Marfan or Ehlers Danlos syndrome, *Am J Obstet Gynecol* 182(5):1021–1023, 2000.

Chiaffarino F, Chatenoud L, Dindelli M, et al: Reproductive factors, family history, occupation and risk of uterovaginal prolapse, *Eur J Obstet Gynecol Reprod Biol* 82(1):63–67, 1999.

Clark AL, Gregory T, Smith VJ, et al: Epidemiologic evaluation of reoperation for surgically treated pelvic organ prolapse and urinary incontinence, *Am J Obstet Gynecol* 189(5):1261–1267, 2003.

Dällenbach P, Kaelin-Gambirasio I, Dubuisson JB, et al: Risk factors for pelvic organ prolapse repair after hysterectomy, *Obstet Gynecol* 110:625–632, 2007.

Delancey JO: The hidden epidemic of pelvic floor dysfunction: achievable goals for improved prevention and treatment, *Am J Obstet Gynecol* 192:1488–1495, 2005.

Dietz HP: The aetiology of prolapse, *Int Urogynecol J Pelvic Floor Dysfunct* 19:1323–1329, 2008.

Dietz HP: Pelvic floor ultrasound: a review, *Am J Obstet Gynecol* 202(4):321–324, 2010.

Handa VL, Garrett E, Hendrix S, et al: Progression and remission of pelvic organ prolapse: a longitudinal study of menopausal women, *Am J Obstet Gynecol* 190(1):27–32, 2004.

Handa VL, Zyczynski HM, Brubaker L, et al: Sexual function before and after sacrocolpopexy for pelvic organ prolapse, *Am J Obstet Gynecol* 197(6):e1–e6, 2007.

Haylen BT, de Ridder D, Freeman RM, et al: An International Urogynecological Association (IUGA)/ International Continence Society (ICS) joint report on the terminology for female pelvic floor dysfunction, *Neurourol Urodyn* 29(1):4–20, 2010.

Hendrix S, Clark A, Nygaard I, et al: Pelvic organ prolapse in the Women's Health Initiative: gravity and gravidity, *Am J Obstet Gynecol* 186:1160–1166, 2002.

Jackson SR, Avery NC, Tarlton JF, et al: Changes in metabolism of collagen in genitourinary prolapse, *Lancet* 347:1658–1661, 1996.

Luber KM, Boero S, Choe JY: The demographics of pelvic floor disorders: current observations and future projections. *Am J Obstet Gynecol* 184:1496–1501, 2001.

Lukacz ES, Lawrence JM, Contreras R, et al: Parity, mode of delivery, and pelvic floor disorder, *Obstet Gynecol* 107(6):1253–1260, 2006.

Mant J, Painter R, Vessey M: Epidemiology of genital prolapse: observation of the Oxford Family Planning Association Study, *Br J Obstet Gynaecol* 104(5):579–585, 1997.

Marchionni M, Bracco GL, Checcucci V, et al: True incidence of vaginal vault prolapse. Thirteen years experience, *J Reprod Med* 44:679–684, 1999.

Miedel A, Tegerstedt G, Maehle-Schmidt M, et al: Nonobstetric risk factors for symptomatic pelvic organ prolapse, *Obstet Gynecol* 113(5):1089–1097, 2009.

Moalli PA, Jones-Ivy S, Meyn LA, et al: Risk factors associated with pelvic floor disorders in women undergoing surgical repair, *Obstet Gynecol* 101:869–874, 2003.

Moalli PA, Shand SH, Zyczneski HM, et al: Remodeling of vaginal connective tissue in patients with prolapse, *Obstet Gynecol* 106:953–963, 2005.

Morley GW, DeLancey JO: Sacrospinous ligament fixation for eversion of the vagina, *Am J Obstet Gynecol* 158:872–881, 1988.

Nygaard I, Bradley C, Brandt D: Women's Health Initiative: Pelvic organ prolapse in older women: prevalence and risk factors, *Obstet Gynecol* 104(3):489–497, 2004.

Nygaard I, Barber MD, Burgio KL, et al: Prevalence of symptomatic pelvic floor disorder in US women, *JAMA* 300(11):1311–1316, 2008.

Olsen AL, Smith VJ, Bergstrom JO, et al: Epidemiology of surgically managed pelvic organ prolapse and urinary incontinence, *Obstet Gynecol* 89(4):501–506, 1997.

Phillips CH, Anthony F, Benyon C, et al: Collagen metabolism in the uterosacral ligaments and vaginal skin in women with uterine prolapse, *BJOG* 113:39–46, 2006.

Rogers RG, Kammerer-Doak D, Villarreal A, et al: A new instrument to measure sexual function in women with urinary incontinence or pelvic organ prolapse, *Am J Obstet Gynecol* 184(4):552–558, 2001.

Rogers RG, Coates KW, Kammerer-Doak D, et al: A short form of the Pelvic Organ Prolapse/Urinary Incontinence Sexual Questionnaire (PISQ-12), *Int Urogynecol J Pelvic Floor Dysfunction* 14(3):164–168, 2003.

Rortveit G, Brown JS, Thom DH, et al: Symptomatic pelvic organ prolapse: prevalence and risk factors in a population-based, racially diverse cohort, *Obstet Gynecol* 109(6):1396–1403, 2007.

Samuelsson EC, Victor FT, Tibblin G, et al: Signs of genital prolapse in a Swedish population of women 20 to 59 years of age and possible related factors. *Am J Obstet Gynecol* 180(2):299–305, 1999.

Schaffer JI, Wai CY, Boreham MK: Etiology of pelvic organ prolapse, *Clin Obstet Gynecol* 48(3):639–647, 2005.

Segev Y, Auslender R, Feiner B, et al: Are women with pelvic organ prolapse at a higher risk of developing hernias? *Int Urogynecol J Pelvic Floor Dysfunct* 20:1451–1453, 2009.

Shah AD, Kohli N, Rajan SS, et al: Racial characteristics of women undergoing surgery for pelvic organ prolapse in the United States, *Am J Obstet Gynecol* 197(1):70.e1–70.e8, 2007.

Silva WA, Pauls RN, Segal JL, et al: Uterosacral ligament vault suspension: five-year outcomes, *Obstet Gynecol* 108:255–263, 2006.

Smith FJ, Holman CD, Moorin RE, et al: Lifetime risk of undergoing surgery for pelvic organ prolapse, *Obstet Gynecol* 116:1096–1100, 2010.

Spence-Jones C, Kamm MA, Henry MM, et al: Bowel-dysfunction: a pathogenetic factor in uterovaginal prolapse and urinary stress incontinence, *Br J Obstet Gynaecol* 101(2):147–152, 1994.

Sung VW, Hampton BS: Epidemiology of pelvic floor dysfunction, *Obstetrics & Gynecology Clinics of North America* 36(3):421–443, 2009.

Sung VW, Washington B, Raker CA: Costs of ambulatory care related to female pelvic floor disorders in the United States, *Am J Obstet Gynecol* 202:483.e1–e4, 2010.

Swift S, Woodman P, O'Boyle A, et al: Pelvic Organ Support Study (POSST): the distribution, clinical definition, and epidemiologic condition of pelvic organ support defects, *Am J Obstet Gynecol* 192(3):795–806, 2005.

Swift SE, Tate SB, Nicholas J: Correlation of symptoms with degree of pelvic organ support in a general population of women: what is pelvic organ prolapse, *Am J Obstet Gynecol* 189(2):372–379, 2003.

Wall LL: The muscles of the pelvic floor, *Clin Obstet Gynecol* 36:910–925, 1993.

Ward KL, Hilton P, UK and Ireland TVT Trial Group: Tension-free vaginal tape versus colposuspension for primary urodynamic stress incontinence: 5-year follow up, *BJOG* 115(2):226–233, 2008.

Whitcomb EL, Rortveit G, Brown JS, et al: Racial differences in pelvic organ prolapse, *Obstet Gynecol* 114(6):1271–1277, 2009.

Withagen MI, Vierhout ME, Milani AL: Does trocar-guided tension-free vaginal mesh (Prolift) repair provoke prolapse of the unaffected compartments? *Int Urogynecol J* 21:271–278, 2010.

Wu JM, Hundley AF, Fulton RG, et al: Forecasting the prevalence of pelvic floor disorders in U.S. Women: 2010 to 2050, *Obstet Gynecol* 114(6):1278–1283, 2009.

Surgical Anatomy of the Pelvis and the Anatomy of Pelvic Support

Mickey Karram MD

 Video Clips online

The reconstructive pelvic surgeon should be familiar with the surgical anatomy of the entire pelvic floor. The goal would be to have a thorough three-dimensional understanding of the anatomy of the vagina, lower urinary tract, and lower gastrointestinal tract, as well as the muscles, nerves, blood vessels, and ligaments that are in the pelvic area. Such an anatomic understanding will facilitate performing procedures in a safe and efficient fashion, allowing the surgeon to access avascular spaces safely, regardless of whether the procedure is being performed vaginally, laparoscopically, or abdominally. The goal of this chapter is to review the surgical anatomy of the pelvis and to describe the anatomy of the various support structures. In addition, a discussion regarding surgical dissection planes is presented.

Anatomy of the Pelvic Floor

The bones of the pelvis provide the foundation to which all of the pelvic structures are ultimately anchored (Figures 2-1 and 2-2). In the standing position, forces are dispersed to minimize the pressures on the pelvic viscera and musculature and to distribute forces to the bones that are better suited for the long-term, cumulative stresses of daily life. In the upright position, the iliopubic rami are oriented in an almost vertical plane. This orientation directs the pressure of the intraabdominal and pelvic contents toward the bones of the pelvis instead of the muscles and endopelvic fascia attachments of the pelvic floor. The pubic rami are nearly horizontal where they articulate in the midline. The weights of the abdominal viscera and some of the pelvic viscera are inferiorly supported by the bony articulation. Numerous ligaments are attached to the pelvic bones, many of which are used in reconstructive pelvic surgery (Figure 2-3).

The pelvic floor is made up of muscular and fascial structures that enclose the abdominal-pelvic cavity, the external vaginal opening, and the urethra and rectum (Figures 2-4 and 2-5). The two types of fascial components are parietal and visceral endopelvic fascia. The parietal fascia covers the pelvic skeletal muscles and provides attachment of muscles to the bony pelvis. It is histologically characterized by regular

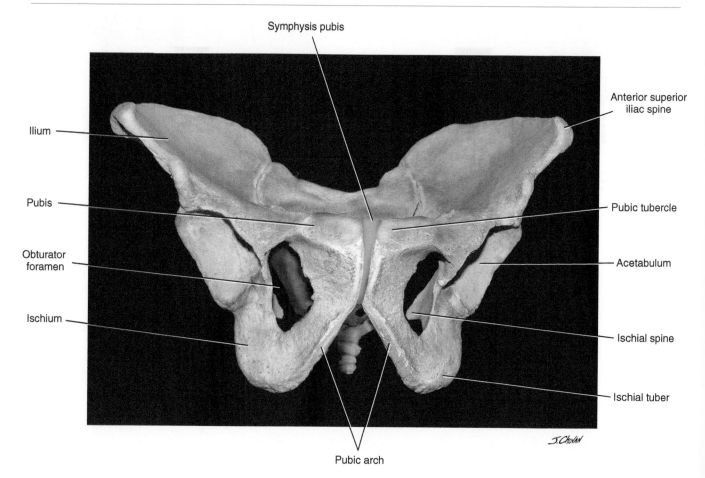

Symphysis pubis

Ilium

Pubis

Obturator
foramen

Ischium

Anterior superior
iliac spine

Pubic tubercle

Acetabulum

Ischial spine

Ischial tuber

Pubic arch

J. Chovan

Figure 2-1 The pelvic bone consists of the ilium, ischium, and pubis. The ilium is bound to the sacrum at the sacroiliac joints. This anterior aspect of the pelvis shows the pubic arch, symphysis, and obturator foramen from a head-on view.

(From Baggish MS, Karram MM: Atlas of pelvic anatomy and gynecologic surgery, *ed 3, St Louis, 2011, Elsevier.)*

arrangements of collagen. Visceral endopelvic fascia is less discrete and exists throughout the pelvis as a mesh network made of loosely arranged collagen, elastin, and adipose tissue, through which blood vessels, lymphatic vessels, and nerves travel to reach the pelvic organs. Examples of visceral endopelvic fascia are discrete ligaments such as the cardinal and uterosacral ligaments. Figure 2-6 demonstrates the relationship of the vagina to other structures in the pelvis and also illustrates how the uterosacral and cardinal ligaments support the upper vagina.

The pelvic side walls are made up of the obturator internus and piriformis muscles. The obturator membrane is a fibrous membrane that covers the obturator foramen (Figure 2-7). The obturator internus originates on the inferior margin of the superior pubic ramus and passes through the lesser sciatic foramen to insert onto the greater trochanter of the femur to rotate the thigh laterally. The piriformis is dorsal and lateral to the coccygeus. It extends from the anterior lateral portion of the sacrum to pass through the greater sciatic foramen and to insert onto the greater trochanter. The pelvic diaphragm consists of the levator ani and coccygeus muscles. The levator ani muscles are divided into the puborectalis, pubococcygeus, and iliococcygeus, which are all skeletal muscles. Other skeletal muscles in the pelvic floor include the external anal sphincter, the striated urethral sphincter, and the superficial perineal muscles (e.g., bulbocavernosus, ischiocavernosus, superficial transverse perinei).

The *pelvic diaphragm* is a term that has been used to describe the hammocklike structure that these muscles create between the pubic bone from the front and the coccyx from behind. The pelvic diaphragm is attached along the lateral pelvic walls to a thickened linear band of obturator fascia called the *arcus tendineus fascia pelvis*. This thickened band forms an identifiable line from the ischial spine to the posterior surface

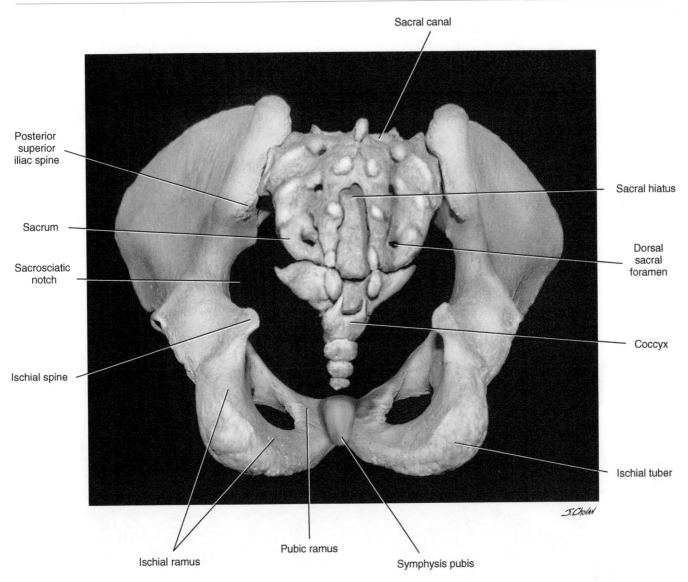

Sacral canal

Posterior superior iliac spine

Sacral hiatus

Sacrum

Dorsal sacral foramen

Sacrosciatic notch

Ischial spine

Coccyx

Ischial tuber

Ischial ramus

Pubic ramus

Symphysis pubis

Figure 2-2 Posterior view of the pelvis is combined with an outlet "looking-in" perspective. The ischial tuberosity, ischial spine, and greater and lesser sacrosciatic notches are best observed from this vantage point. Posterior sacrum highlights include the sacral hiatus, sacral canal, and posterior sacral foramina.

(From Baggish MS, Karram MM: Atlas of pelvic anatomy and gynecologic surgery, *ed 3, St Louis, 2011, Elsevier.)*

of the ipsilateral symphysis pubis. The puborectalis portion of the levator ani originates on the posterior inferior pubic ramus and arcus and passes posteriorly, forming a sling around the vagina, rectum, and perineal body to form the anorectal angle. Some muscle fibers may blend with the muscularis of the vagina, rectum, and external anal sphincter (see Figure 2-5). The pubococcygeus has a similar origin but inserts in the midline onto the anococcygeal raphe and the anterolateral borders of the coccyx. The iliococcygeus originates along the arcus tendineus from the back of the pubis to the ischial spine and inserts on the anococcygeal raphe to form the levator plate. The space through which the rectum, vagina, and urethra pass is called the *genital hiatus* (see Figure 2-7). The coccygeus muscle, who some would consider as part of the levator ani complex, makes up the posterior part of the pelvic floor and also plays a role in support. It originates on the ischial spine, overlies the sacrospinous ligament, and inserts on the lateral lower sacrum and coccyx. As one ages, the coccygeus becomes thinner and more fibrous, often blending with the sacrospinous ligament. At times, distinguishing the two is difficult because of the fact that they have the same origin and insertion. The coccygeus sacrospinous ligament complex (C-SSL) is a very common anchoring point for a variety of prolapse repairs that are discussed and illustrated throughout this text. Appreciating

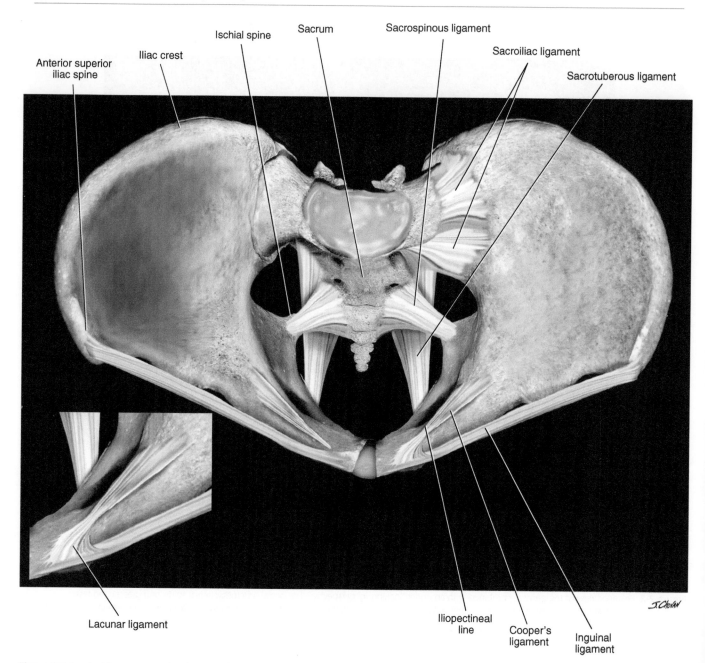

Anterior superior iliac spine

Iliac crest

Ischial spine

Sacrum

Sacrospinous ligament

Sacroiliac ligament

Sacrotuberous ligament

Lacunar ligament

Iliopectineal line

Cooper's ligament

Inguinal ligament

J.Chovan

Figure 2-3 Inguinal ligament stretches between the anterior superior iliac spine and the pubic tubercle. From the latter is reflected the lacunar ligament, which forms the medial boundary of the femoral canal. Cooper ligament is a stout structure that clings to the iliopectineal line *(see inset)*. Between the ischial spines and the lateral aspect of the sacrum is the sacrospinous ligament. This ligament also creates the greater and lesser sacrosciatic foramina.

(From Baggish MS, Karram MM: Atlas of pelvic anatomy and gynecologic surgery, ed 3, St Louis, 2011, Elsevier.)

the close proximity of the many vascular structures and nerves to the C-SSL is extremely important (Figure 2-8). Posterior to the complex are the gluteus maximus muscle and the ischiorectal fossa. The pudendal nerves and vessels lie directly posterior to the ischial spine, and the sciatic nerve lies superior and lateral to the ischial spine. An abundant vascular supply, which includes the inferior gluteal and the hypogastric venous plexus, also lies superior to the ischial spine. The C-SSL complex can be exposed via a posterior perirectal dissection, as well as by anterior paravaginal dissection. The ability of the surgeon to palpate and identify this structure safely is mandatory to avoid significant bleeding or nerve damage.

From a functional standpoint, the levator ani muscle exhibits a constant baseline tone and can also be voluntarily contracted. The muscle contains both Type 1 (slow-twitch) fibers to maintain constant tone and Type II (fast-twitch) fibers to provide reflex

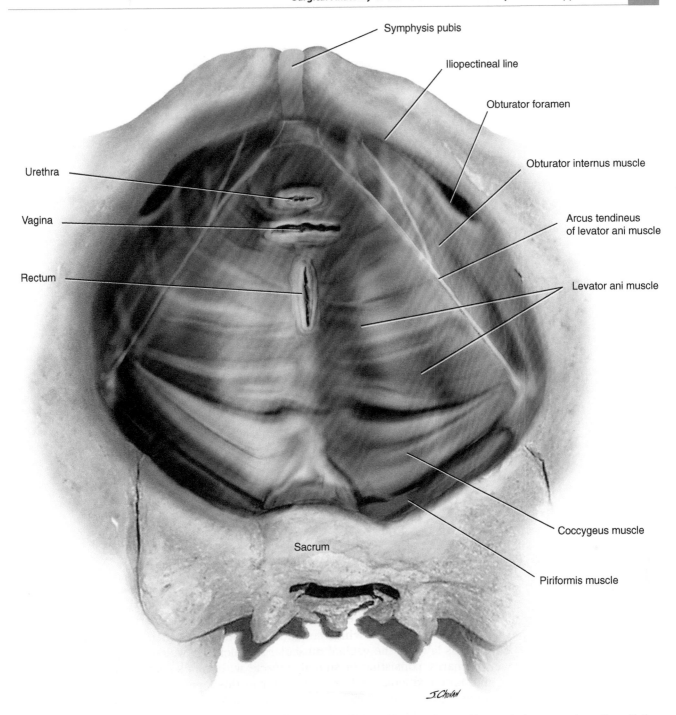

Symphysis pubis

Iliopectineal line

Obturator foramen

Obturator internus muscle

Arcus tendineus
of levator ani muscle

Levator ani muscle

Coccygeus muscle

Piriformis muscle

Sacrum

Urethra

Vagina

Rectum

J.Chovan

Figure 2-4 Intact levator ani muscle is arising along the length of the arcus tendineus. The exposed retropubic space is demonstrated, together with the cut edges of the urethra and vagina.

(From Baggish MS, Karram MM: Atlas of pelvic anatomy and gynecologic surgery, ed 3, St Louis, 2011, Elsevier.)

and voluntary contractions. Constant tone of the pelvic floor, except when voiding or defecating or when intraabdominal pressure is increased, provides a constant support for the pelvic viscera.

Anatomy of the Vagina

The vagina is a hollow fibromuscular tube with rugal folds that extends from the vestibule to the uterine cervix or vaginal apex. In the standing position, the upper two-thirds portion of the vagina is almost horizontal, whereas the lower one third is nearly

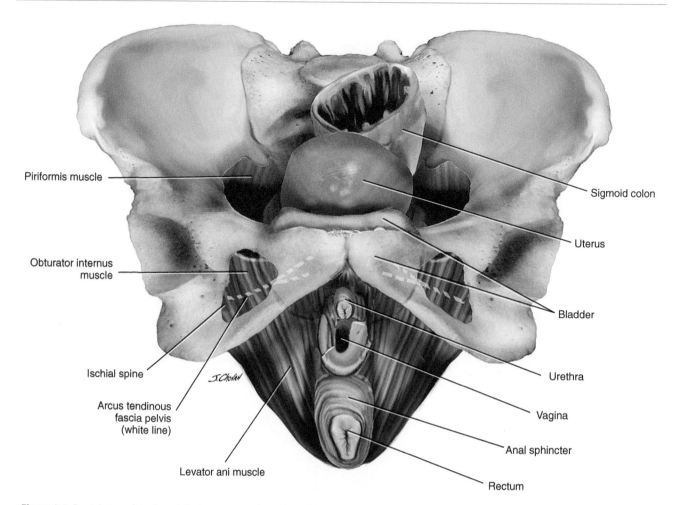

Piriformis muscle

Sigmoid colon

Uterus

Obturator internus
muscle

Bladder

Ischial spine

J.Chovan

Urethra

Arcus tendinous
fascia pelvis
(white line)

Vagina

Anal sphincter

Levator ani muscle

Rectum

Figure 2-5 Frontal view of the funnel-like levator ani and its relationship to the vulva and superficial muscles of the perineum are illustrated. The levator arises, in part, from the inferior margins of the pubic bone. The artist has superimposed the arcus tendineus *(dashed white line)* onto the obturator internus and pubic bone.

(From Baggish MS, Karram MM: Atlas of pelvic anatomy and gynecologic surgery, *ed 3, St Louis, 2011, Elsevier.)*

vertical. The vaginal wall is composed of three layers. It is lined by nonkeratinizing stratified squamous epithelium that lies over a thin, loose layer of connective tissue, called the *lamina propria,* which contains no glands but contains small blood vessels. Beneath this layer is the vaginal muscularis, which is a well-developed fibromuscular layer, primarily consisting of smooth muscle with smaller amounts of collagen and elastin. Many textbooks and surgeons refer to this layer as *fascia.* The muscularis is surrounded by an adventitial layer, which is a variably discrete layer of collagen, elastin, and adipose tissue containing blood vessels, lymphatic vessels, and nerves. The adventitia represents an extension of the visceral endopelvic fascia that surrounds the vagina and is adjacent to the bladder and rectum. This layer allows for the independent expansion and contraction of these visceral organs. The walls of the vagina are in direct contact with each other except where its lumen is held open by the cervix. Surgical terms, such as *pubocervical fascia* and *rectovaginal fascia,* refer to layers that are developed as a result of separating the vaginal epithelium from the muscularis or by splitting the vaginal muscularis layer. The proximate and midportions of the anterior vaginal wall support the bladder base, being separated from the vesicovaginal adventia (endopelvic fascia). The urethra is fused to the distal anterior vagina with a nondistinct adventitial layer separating them. The terminal portions of the ureters cross that lateral fornices of the vagina on their way to the bladder base (Figure 2-9). **(See Video 2-1, "Surgical Anatomy of the Anterior Vaginal Wall."**)

The vagina is related posteriorly to the cul-de-sac and rectal ampulla and is related inferiorly to the perineal body. The connective tissue of the perineal body extends 2

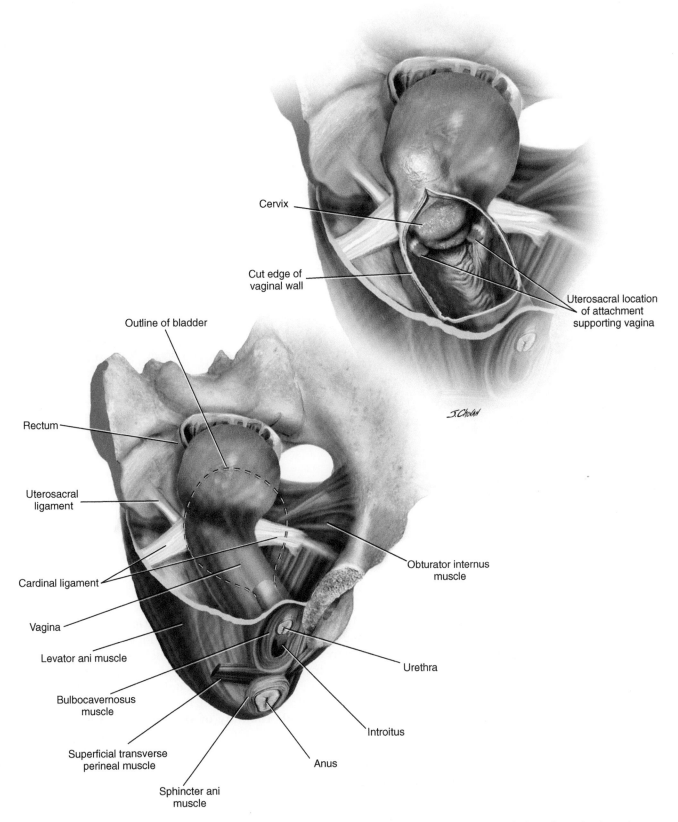

Cervix

Cut edge of
vaginal wall

Uterosacral location
of attachment
supporting vagina

J. Chovan

Outline of bladder

Rectum

Uterosacral
ligament

Cardinal ligament

Vagina

Levator ani muscle

Bulbocavernosus
muscle

Superficial transverse
perineal muscle

Sphincter ani
muscle

Anus

Introitus

Urethra

Obturator internus
muscle

Figure 2-6 This three-dimensional drawing illustrates the relationship of the vagina to other structures in the pelvis. The lower figure also shows the superimposed outline of the urinary bladder, relative to the vagina. The upper vagina shares support with the uterus and bladder. Principally, the upper vagina consists of the deep cardinal ligament and, to a lesser extent, the uterosacral ligaments. In the upper illustration, the schematically drawn location of a portion of the uterosacral ligaments is attached to the vagina. The lower vagina is clearly supported by the levator ani muscle, anal sphincter, and deep vascular structures located beneath the bulbocavernosus muscle, as well as by the commonly shared connective tissue, smooth muscle, and vessels found in the tissues between the rectum and vagina and, likewise, between the bladder and vagina. Between these anchors, the lateral vaginal wall is not attached and opens into a fat-filled paravaginal space. If the lateral wall is cut and the fat being dissected is removed, then the anatomist will be looking into a retropubic (extraperitoneal) space filled with fat. If the fat is cleaned away, the obturator internus muscle is visible.

(From Baggish MS, Karram MM: Atlas of pelvic anatomy and gynecologic surgery, ed 3, St Louis, 2011, Elsevier.)

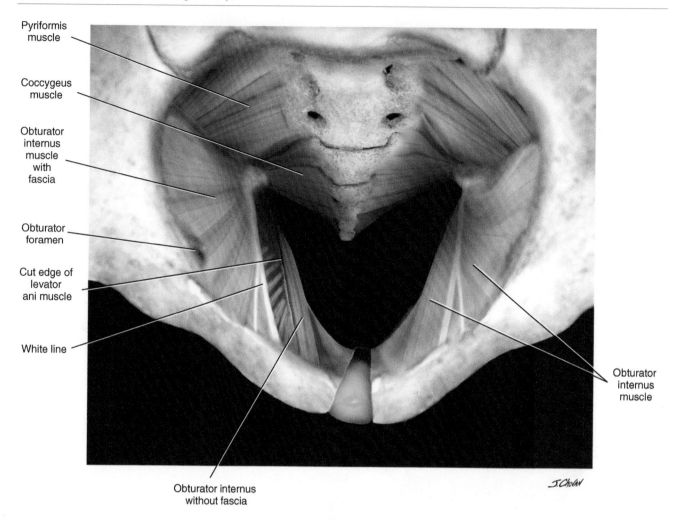

Pyriformis muscle

Coccygeus muscle

Obturator internus muscle with fascia

Obturator foramen

Cut edge of levator ani muscle

White line

Obturator internus muscle

Obturator internus without fascia

J.Chovan

Figure 2-7 The large obturator internus muscle covered with tough obturator fascia forms the pelvic sidewall. The arcus tendineus, or white line, is produced by a thickened area of obturator fascia. The levator ani muscle arises from the arcus. The cut edge of the levator is shown on the patient's right side (viewer's left side). The left levator has been removed. The piriformis and coccygeus muscles complete the enclosure of the pelvis.

(From Baggish MS, Karram MM: Atlas of pelvic anatomy and gynecologic surgery, *ed 3, St Louis, 2011, Elsevier.)*

to 3 cm cephalad from the hymenal ring along the posterior vaginal wall and forms what has been called the *rectovaginal fascia*. As previously mentioned, these terms have been recently debated, and many surgical anatomists have concluded that between the adjacent organs is primarily vaginal muscularis with no fascia being histologically present. Mobilization and plication of this tissue is how a defect-specific rectocele procedure is performed. (See Chapter 9, "Surgical Correction of Posterior Pelvic Floor Defects." **See also Video 2-2, "Surgical Anatomy of the Posterior Vaginal Wall."** 📣)

Anatomy of the Perineum

The perineum is divided into superficial and deep components. These two components are separated by a fibrous connective tissue layer called the *perineal membrane*, which is a triangular sheet of dense fibromuscular tissue that spans the entire path of the pelvic outlet. It has also been sometimes referred to as the *urogenital diaphragm*. The perineal membrane provides support to the distal vagina and urethra as they pass through it. The deep perineal compartment is composed of the deep transverse perineal muscle; portions of the external urethral sphincter muscles,

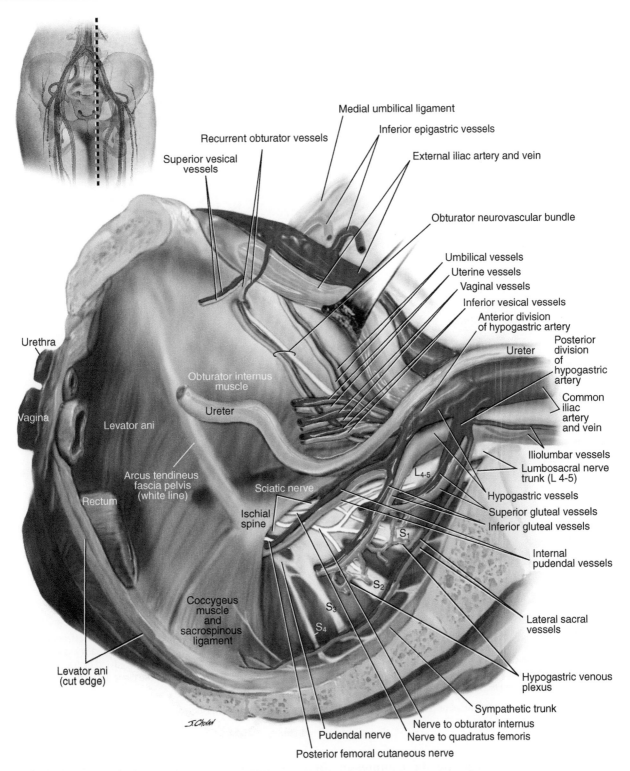

Medial umbilical ligament

Recurrent obturator vessels

Inferior epigastric vessels

Superior vesical vessels

External iliac artery and vein

Obturator neurovascular bundle

Umbilical vessels

Uterine vessels

Vaginal vessels

Inferior vesical vessels

Anterior division of hypogastric artery

Ureter

Posterior division of hypogastric artery

Common iliac artery and vein

Urethra

Obturator internus muscle

Vagina

Ureter

Levator ani

Iliolumbar vessels

Lumbosacral nerve trunk (L 4-5)

L₄₋₅

Arcus tendineus fascia pelvis (white line)

Sciatic nerve

Hypogastric vessels

Superior gluteal vessels

Inferior gluteal vessels

Rectum

Ischial spine

S₁

Internal pudendal vessels

Coccygeus muscle and sacrospinous ligament

S₂

S₃

S₄

Lateral sacral vessels

Levator ani (cut edge)

Hypogastric venous plexus

Sympathetic trunk

Nerve to obturator internus

Pudendal nerve

Nerve to quadratus femoris

Posterior femoral cutaneous nerve

Figure 2-8 Sagittal section through the pelvis *(inset)*. The muscles enclosing the pelvis include the sidewall muscles; that is, the obturator internus, coccygeus, and piriformis. The white line, or arcus tendineus, stretches between the ischial spine and the lower margin of the pubic bone. The levator ani takes its origin from the thickened obturator internus fascia (the arcus tendineus), as well as from the lower margin of the pubic ramus. The bifurcation of the common iliac vessels is demonstrated. The internal iliac, or hypogastric, vessels supply the pelvic viscera via several branches and tributaries. The hypogastric artery divides into the superoposterior and inferoanterior divisions. From the posterior division, the superior gluteal, lateral sacral, and iliolumbar vessels emanate. The anterior division includes the lateral umbilical, superior and inferior vesicles, obturator, uterine, and vaginal branches. Terminal branches of the anterior division include the inferior gluteal and internal pudendal vessels. The posterior division of the hypogastric artery will lead the dissector to the sacral nerve roots and sciatic nerve. The obturator neurovascular bundle is best exposed by the retraction of the external iliac vein. The lateral umbilical vessels ascend the anterior abdominal wall, supported superficially to the external iliac vessels on either side of the urachus *(not shown here)*.

(From Baggish MS, Karram MM: Atlas of pelvic anatomy and gynecologic surgery, ed 3, St Louis, 2011, Elsevier.)

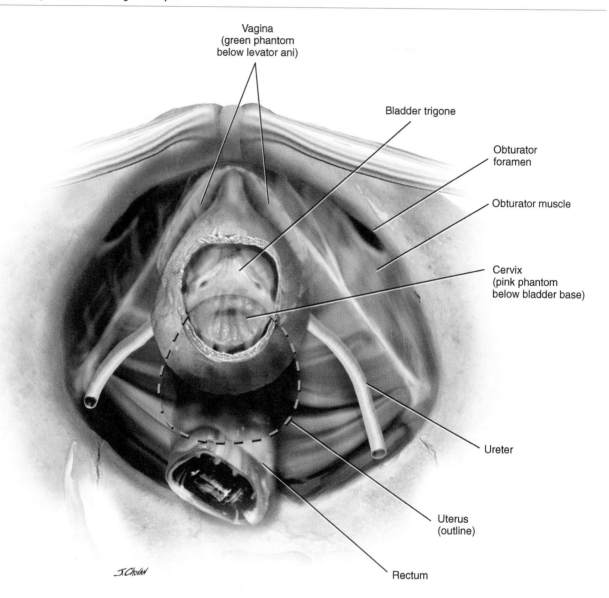

Figure 2-9 Full frontal view of the bladder with an anterior window of tissue excised shows the trigone and interureteric ridge. Posteriorly beneath the bladder lies the (phantom) uterus and cervix *(pink)*. The bladder base overlies the cervix and vagina *(green)*. The phantom vagina is visualized because this stylized drawing has presumed to make the posterior wall of the bladder selectively transparent. A misplaced and high suture is placed in the vagina during a colposuspension, which could injure the terminal ureter. The ureters must traverse the tissue above the anterolateral vaginal fornices to reach the bladder.

(From Baggish MS, Karram MM: Atlas of pelvic anatomy and gynecologic surgery, *ed 3, St Louis, 2011, Elsevier.)*

which are the compressor urethrae; and the urethrovaginal sphincter and portions of the external anal sphincter, as well as the vaginal musculofascial attachments. The neurovascular anatomy of the perineum is illustrated in Figure 2-10. The motor and sensory innervation of the perineum is via the pudendal nerve. The pudendal nerve originates from S_2 to S_4 and exits the pelvis through the greater sciatic foramen, hooks around the ischial spine, and then travels along the medial surface of the obturator internus and through the ischiorectal fossa in a thickening of fascia called *Alcock canal*. It emerges posteriorly and medially to the ischial tuberosity and divides into three branches—the clitoral, perineal, and inferior rectal nerves. The blood supply to the perineum is from the pudendal artery, which travels with the pudendal nerve.

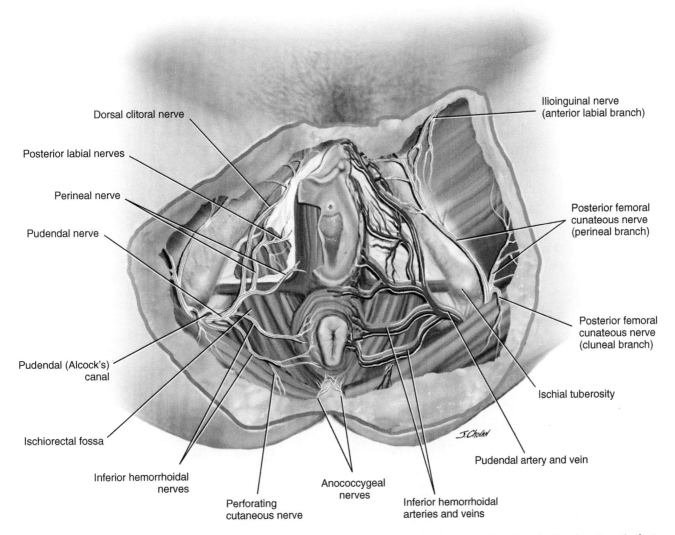

Dorsal clitoral nerve

Posterior labial nerves

Perineal nerve

Pudendal nerve

Pudendal (Alcock's) canal

Ischiorectal fossa

Inferior hemorrhoidal nerves

Perforating cutaneous nerve

Anococcygeal nerves

Inferior hemorrhoidal arteries and veins

Ilioinguinal nerve (anterior labial branch)

Posterior femoral cunateous nerve (perineal branch)

Posterior femoral cunateous nerve (cluneal branch)

Ischial tuberosity

Pudendal artery and vein

J.Chován

Figure 2-10 Pudendal nerves and internal pudendal vessels emerge from the Alcock canal just medial to the ischial tuberosity. Branches pierce the fascia covering the muscles and can be found with the perineal fat. Colles fascia has largely been stripped away in this drawing.

(From Baggish MS, Karram MM: Atlas of pelvic anatomy and gynecologic surgery, ed 3, St Louis, 2011, Elsevier.)

Transobturator, Inner Groin, and Retropubic Anatomy

With the popularity of synthetic slings and trocal-based mesh kits, a thorough understanding of the anatomy of the obturator membrane, retropubic space, and muscles of the inner thigh is of extreme importance (Figure 2-11). The obturator membrane is a fibrous sheath that spans the obturator foramen, through which the obturator neurovascular bundle penetrates via the obturator canal. The obturator artery and vein originate as branches of the internal iliac vessels. These vessels exit the lower pelvis by traveling through the retropubic space and entering the obturator canal. As they emerge from the inferior side of the obturator membrane and enter the obturator space, they divide into many small branches supplying the muscles of the adductor compartment of the thigh. The vessels are predominantly small (usually less than 5 mm in diameter) and splinter into variable courses. The muscles of the medial thigh and adductor compartment from superficial to deep are the following: gracilis, adductor longus, adductor brevis, adductor magnus, and obturator externus muscles (Figure 2-12). The obturator nerve emerges from the obturator membrane and bifurcates into anterior and posterior divisions, traveling distally down the thigh to supply the muscles of the adductor compartment. With the patient in the dorsal lithotomy position, the nerves and vessels follow the thigh and laterally course away from the ischiopubic ramus and are nicely

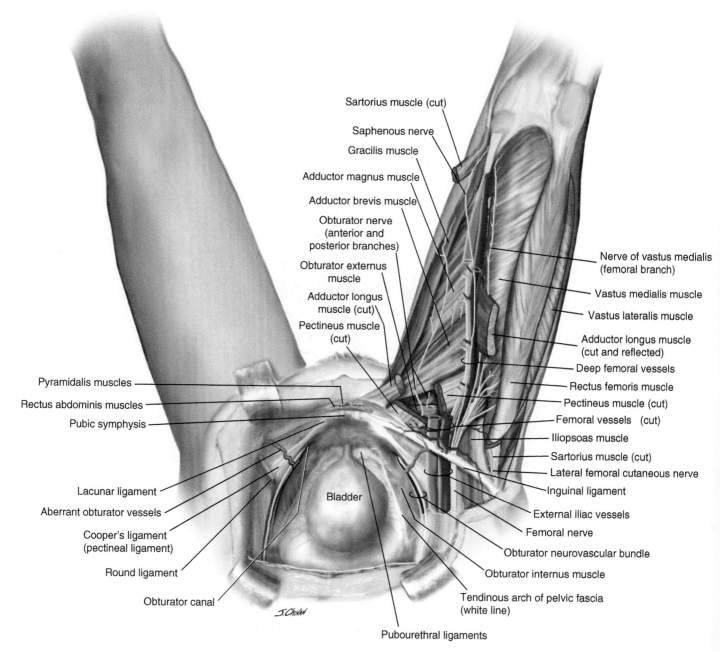

Sartorius muscle (cut)

Saphenous nerve

Gracilis muscle

Adductor magnus muscle

Adductor brevis muscle

Obturator nerve (anterior and posterior branches)

Obturator externus muscle

Adductor longus muscle (cut)

Pectineus muscle (cut)

Pyramidalis muscles

Rectus abdominis muscles

Pubic symphysis

Lacunar ligament

Aberrant obturator vessels

Cooper's ligament (pectineal ligament)

Round ligament

Obturator canal

Bladder

Nerve of vastus medialis (femoral branch)

Vastus medialis muscle

Vastus lateralis muscle

Adductor longus muscle (cut and reflected)

Deep femoral vessels

Rectus femoris muscle

Pectineus muscle (cut)

Femoral vessels (cut)

Iliopsoas muscle

Sartorius muscle (cut)

Lateral femoral cutaneous nerve

Inguinal ligament

External iliac vessels

Femoral nerve

Obturator neurovascular bundle

Obturator internus muscle

Tendinous arch of pelvic fascia (white line)

Pubourethral ligaments

Figure 2-11 Anatomy of the retropubic space is it relates to the thigh.

(From Baggish MS, Karram MM: Atlas of pelvic anatomy and gynecologic surgery, ed 3, St Louis, 2011, Elsevier.)

protected by the tendon of the adductor longus. **(See Videos 2-3, 2-4, and 2-5 to view this anatomy on cadaveric specimens and live patients. 📹)**

Anatomy of the Lower Urinary Tract

The female urethra is approximately 4 cm long and averages 6 mm in diameter. Its lumen is slightly curved as it passes from the retropubic space, perforates the perineal membrane, and ends with its external orifice in the vestibule directly above the vaginal opening. Throughout its length, the urethra is embedded in the adventitia of the anterior vaginal wall.

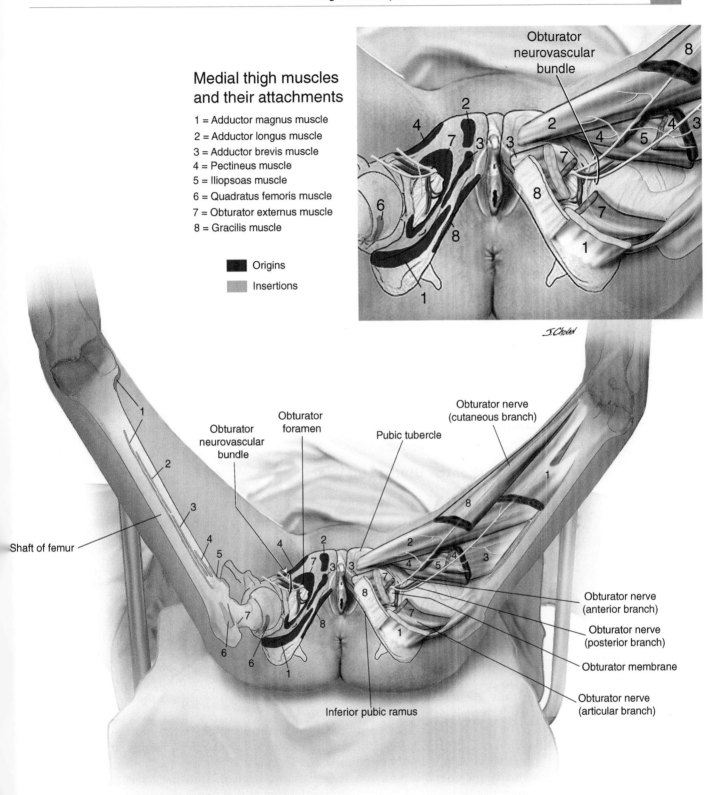

Medial thigh muscles and their attachments

1 = Adductor magnus muscle
2 = Adductor longus muscle
3 = Adductor brevis muscle
4 = Pectineus muscle
5 = Iliopsoas muscle
6 = Quadratus femoris muscle
7 = Obturator externus muscle
8 = Gracilis muscle

■ Origins

■ Insertions

Obturator neurovascular bundle

J.Chovan

Shaft of femur

Obturator neurovascular bundle

Obturator foramen

Pubic tubercle

Obturator nerve (cutaneous branch)

Obturator nerve (anterior branch)

Obturator nerve (posterior branch)

Obturator membrane

Obturator nerve (articular branch)

Inferior pubic ramus

Figure 2-12 Illustration of the anatomy of the inner thigh. The origins and insertion of medial thigh muscles are demonstrated.

From Baggish MS, Karram MM: Atlas of pelvic anatomy and gynecologic surgery, ed 3, St Louis, 2011, Elsevier.)

The bladder is a hollow muscular organ that is the reservoir for the urinary system. The anterior bladder is extraperitoneally adjacent to the retropubic space or Retzius space. The bladder rests inferiorly on the anterior vagina and lower uterine segment, separated by an envelope of adventitia or endopelvic fascia. The bladder wall musculature is often described as having three layers—the inner longitudinal, middle circular, and outer longitudinal layers. However, this layering occurs only at the bladder neck; the remainder of the bladder musculature is made up of fibers that run in many directions, both within and among the layers.

The trigone is a triangular area in the bladder base and has a flattened appearance with a smooth epithelial covering. The corners of the trigone are formed by three orifices—the paired ureteral orifices and the internal urethral orifice. The superior boundary of the trigone is a slightly raised area between the two ureteral orifices called the *interureteric ridge*. The two ureteral openings are slitlike, are in an undistended bladder, and lie approximately 3 cm apart.

The ureter travels retroperitoneally from the renal pelvis to the bladder and is anatomically divided into abdominal and pelvic segments that are approximately equal in length, 12 to 15 cm each. The ureter enters the pelvis by crossing over the iliac vessels where the common iliac artery divides into the external iliac and hypogastric vessels. The ureter travels lateral to the hypogastric artery and is attached to the peritoneum of the lateral pelvic side wall.

As the ureter proceeds more distally, it courses along the lateral side of the uterosacral ligament and enters the endopelvic fascia of the parametrium. The ureter courses medially toward the uterosacral ligament as it travels from the sacrum toward the vagina. At the level of the ischial spine, the ureter is approximately 2.3 cm lateral to the uterosacral ligament. The ureter is closest to the uterosacral ligament at its distal end, where it is approximately 1 cm lateral to the ligament. The ureter then moves medially over the lateral vaginal fornix and travels through the wall of the bladder until it reaches the trigone. The distal part of the ureter is the most common site of injury during gynecologic and reconstructive procedures. Figure 2-13 illustrates the anatomy of the lowest portion of the ureter. **(See Video 2-6, "Anatomy of the Bladder and Lower Ureter," for a demonstration of this anatomy on a cadaver.**

Support of the Uterus and Vagina

Normal pelvic support is provided by an interaction between the pelvic floor muscles and the connective tissue attachments. The primary support of the pelvic floor comes from the pelvic muscles, which provide a firm yet elastic base on which the pelvic organs rest. The pelvic organs are stabilized in an appropriate position by the endopelvic fascia or connective tissue. During micturition or defecation, the pelvic floor muscles will relax while the connective tissue attachments temporarily stabilize the pelvic organs.

The endopelvic fascia is best described as a network of loose connective tissue that surrounds the pelvic organs and loosely connects them to the supportive musculature and pelvic bones. The endopelvic fascia provides stabilization and some support, but it also allows for mobility, expansion, and contraction of the viscera to permit storage and evacuation of urine and stool, as well as appropriate coitus and parturition. Histologically, the endopelvic fascia is made up of collagen, elastin, adipose tissue, nerves, vessels, lymph channels, and smooth muscle.

The uterus does not have any fixed supports other than the support provided at the level of the cervix. This is indicated by its ability to enlarge without restriction during pregnancy. As previously mentioned, the upper two thirds portion of the vagina is in a nearly horizontal orientation in a standing woman. DeLancey has described how connective tissue attachments stabilize the vagina at different levels (DeLancey, 1992). Level 1 supports the upper vagina and cervix by the uterosacral-cardinal ligament complex. Level II supports the paravaginal attachments along the length of the vagina to the arcus tendineus fascia pelvis or to the white line anteriorly and pararectally into the levator ani muscle posteriorly. Level III support describes the most inferior or distal portions of the vagina, including the perineum. Remembering that all three levels of support are connected through the continuation of the endopelvic fascia is important.

Level I support of the cervix and upper vagina maintains vaginal length and keeps the vaginal axis nearly horizontal, so that it rests on the rectum. This position allows

Figure 2-13 The ureter enters the upper portion of the cardinal ligament, which consists of condensed fat and fibrous tissue and is honeycombed with venous sinuses. The ureter passes beneath the bladder pillar (vesicouterine ligament) to enter the base of the urinary bladder obliquely (trigone).

(From Baggish MS, Karram MM: Atlas of pelvic anatomy and gynecologic surgery, ed 3, St Louis, 2011, Elsevier.)

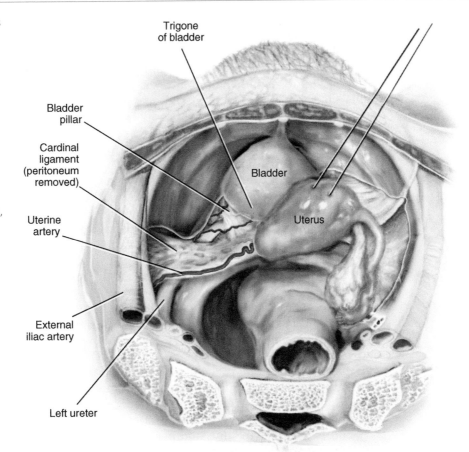

Trigone of bladder

Bladder pillar

Cardinal ligament (peritoneum removed)

Bladder

Uterine artery

Uterus

External iliac artery

Left ureter

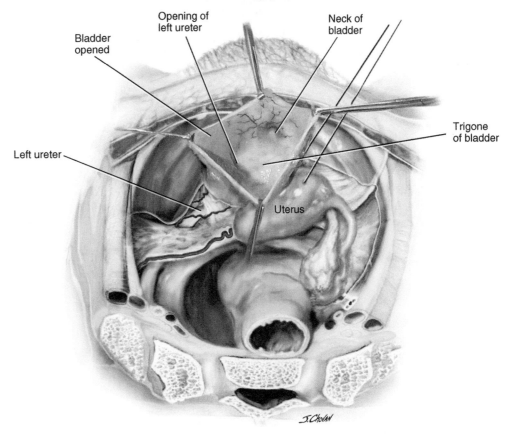

Opening of left ureter

Bladder opened

Neck of bladder

Left ureter

Trigone of bladder

Uterus

J. Chovan

the cervix to stay superior to the level of the ischial spine. At this level the cervix and cardinal ligaments blend with the uterosacral ligaments and are difficult to delineate precisely from one another. Fibers traveling predominantly toward the sacrum make up the uterosacral ligaments, whereas those traveling predominantly in a lateral direction make up the cardinal ligaments (see Figure 2-9). Together, the fibers form a three-dimensional complex attaching the upper vagina and cervix to the sacrum and lateral sacral sidewalls at the level of the coccygeus muscle, levator ani, piriformis, and possibly even the obturator internus fascia that overlies the ischial spine. **(See Video 2-7, "Anatomy of the Uterosacral Ligament," to view the anatomy of the uterosacral ligament on a live patient.** 📹**)**

Level II support functions to keep the vagina in a midline position directly over the rectum. As previously mentioned, the arcus or white line is a thickened condensation of the parietal fascia in which the paravaginal endopelvic fascia connects, supporting the vagina and creating the anterior lateral vaginal sulci. The arcus originates at the level of the ischial spine and inserts on the inferior aspect of the superior pubic rami over the origin of the puborectalis muscle. Similar to the anterior paravaginal support, posterior lateral supports are also present. The endopelvic fascia extends posteriorly from the posterior lateral vaginal sulci around the rectum to attach the vagina to the pelvic floor. These fibers blend anteriorly with the vaginal muscularis, posteriorly with the rectal muscularis, and inferiorly with the perineal body.

Level III support is provided by the perineal body, perineal membrane, superficial and deep perineal muscles, and endopelvic fascia. These structures support and maintain the normal position of the distal one third of the vagina and introitus. The separation of the perineal body from the perineal membrane can result in perineal descent, which can potentially contribute to defecatory dysfunction. Figure 2-14 illustrates the three levels of support as described by DeLancey (DeLancey, 1992).

When the vagina, rectum, and bladder are kept in the horizontal plane over the levator plate and pelvic floor muscles and intraabdominal and gravitational forces are applied perpendicularly to the vagina, the pelvic floor musculature counters these forces with its constant tone. This horizontal position and support by the levator ani

Figure 2-14 Three levels of support as described by DeLancey.

(From DeLancey JOL: Anatomic aspects of vaginal eversion after hysterectomy, Am J Obstet Gynecol 166:1717–1724, 1992.)

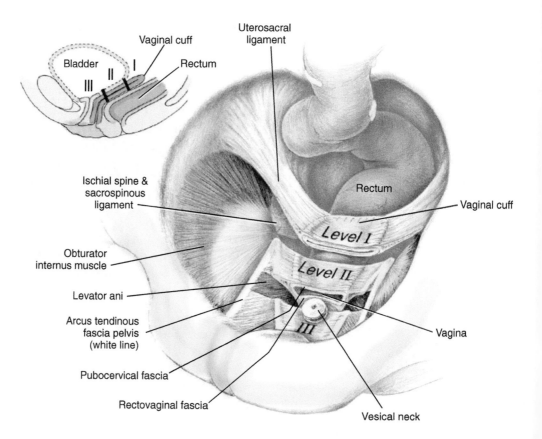

maintain pelvic organ support. Further, in times of acute stress, such as a cough or a sneeze, a reflex contraction of the pelvic floor musculature counters and further stabilizes the viscera. The genital hiatus also responds to these acute forces by narrowing to maintain level III support. When the pelvic floor weakens, such as with obvious neurologic injury or long-standing mechanical damage, the endopelvic fascia can become the primary mechanism of support. If the endopelvic fascia attachments break down, the result is stretching or attenuation of endopelvic fascia support, resulting in changes in vector forces applied to the viscera, leading to pelvic organ prolapse with or without visceral dysfunction. The re-creation of these supportive connections and the proper positioning of the organs without significant alteration of the vaginal axis, thus maintaining adequate vaginal length, should be the goals of any reconstructive surgical procedure.

Surgical Dissection Planes

When performing reconstructive pelvic surgery, whether transvaginally, abdominally, or laparoscopically, the surgeon must have a clear understanding of the appropriate surgical planes. Avascular dissection planes are present throughout the pelvic floor and are, at times, even more prominent in the presence of pelvic organ prolapse. A number of avascular planes or spaces retroperitoneally exist within the pelvis, which can be valuable to the pelvic surgeon. These spaces lack blood vessels and nerves and are filled with loose areolar tissue that allow, when appropriate, blunt dissection. The pelvic reconstructive surgeon should be familiar with these spaces, as well as their relationships with one another. Such an anatomic understanding will help avoid injury to the viscera and vasculature, restore normal anatomic relationships in the case of distorted anatomy, and resect pelvic disease such as adhesion formation, pelvic infection, endometriosis, or cancer, as well as a foreign body such as synthetic mesh. These spaces include the vesicovaginal space and the paravesical, pararectal, rectovaginal, prevesical (or retropubic), and presacral spaces (Figure 2-15). These dissection planes are surgically relevant when dissecting the bladder away from the anterior vaginal wall and the rectum away from the posterior vaginal wall. Appropriate dissection and identification of the preperitoneal space, which leads to the anterior and posterior cul-de-sac, are of extreme importance when performing a vaginal hysterectomy, especially in the patient with an elongated cervix or when isolating an enterocele sac in the patient with posthysterectomy prolapse.

When performing an anterior or posterior vaginal wall incision as part of a prolapse repair, the depth of the incision determines the anatomic plane that is developed. Specifically, an incision made superficially creates a plane between the vaginal epithelium and the fibromuscular part of the vaginal wall. Deeper incisions can result in splitting the fibromuscular layer or even result in a plane deep to the fibromuscular layer, which would be the true vesicovaginal or rectovaginal space.

When performing a dissection of the anterior vaginal wall, the surgeon should be familiar with the fact that the distal most portion of the anterior vaginal wall is fused to the posterior urethra. This anatomic relationship is extremely important when performing a synthetic midurethral sling. The dissection of the vagina off the posterior urethra must be sharply performed, since no clear plane differentiates these two structures. As the vaginal incision proceeds in a proximal direction, the dissection plane between the anterior vaginal wall and the proximal urethra and bladder base becomes more apparent; allowing, the vagina to be peeled off the bladder in a relatively avascular fashion **(see Video 2-1)**.

In the author's opinion, the extent of dissection of the anterior vaginal wall when performing a cystocele repair should be to the lateral pelvic sidewall or to the inferior pubic ramus on each side to determine whether lateral paravaginal support is present. In addition, the base of the bladder should be proximally dissected to the level of the vesicouterine space to determine whether an enterocele sac is present in the patient who has undergone a hysterectomy or to mobilize completely the base of the bladder off the cervix in a patient with a uterus.

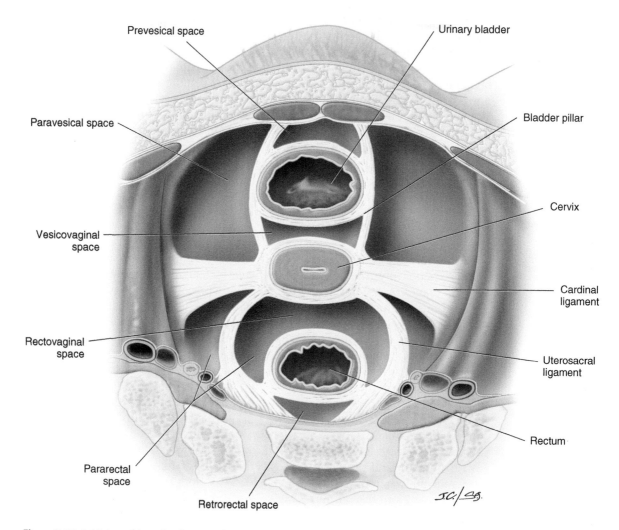

Figure 2-15 Axial view of the pelvis illustrates the avascular spaces within the pelvis.

(From Walters MD, Barber MD: Hysterectomy for benign disease. In Karram M, editor: Female pelvic surgery video atlas series, *Philadelphia, 2010, Elsevier.)*

Such a dissection allows for the complete mobilization of the bladder off the vagina and surrounding structures, as well as allows for the safe passage of any sling material or other instruments or meshes that may be needed to repair the prolapse.

Regarding the dissection of the posterior vaginal wall off the anterior wall of the rectum, the surgeon should be aware of the fact that the distal portion of the posterior vagina maintains its support via connective tissue that extends approximately 3 cm cephalad from the perineum. In the author's opinion, a dissection of the posterior vaginal wall in a patient with prolapse should extend laterally to the level of the levator fascia and proximally to a point above the extraperitoneal portion of the rectum. Such a dissection will completely mobilize the anterior wall of the rectum off the posterior vaginal wall and allow for the identification of a co-existent posterior or apical enterocele.

SUMMARY: A clear and thorough understanding of pelvic floor anatomy is mandatory before performing pelvic reconstructive procedures in women with pelvic organ prolapse. The surgeon should approach every case with a clear surgical plan that addresses the level and extent of dissection that will be required to complete the planned procedure safely.

Suggested Readings

Baggish MS, Karram MM: *Atlas of pelvic anatomy and gynecologic surgery*, ed 3, St Louis, 2010, Elsevier.

Barber MD, Bremer RE, Thor KB, et al: Innervation of the female lavatory ani muscles, *Am J Obstet Gynecol* 187:64–71, 2002.

Buller JL, Thompson JR, Cundiff GW, et al: Uterosacral ligament: description of anatomic relationships to optimize surgical safety, *Obstet Gynecol* 97:873–879, 2001.

Campbell RM: The anatomy and histology of the sacrouterine ligaments, *Am J Obstet Gynecol* 59:1–12, 1950.

DeLancey JOL: Correlative study of paraurethral anatomy, *Obstet Gynecol* 68:91–97, 1986.

DeLancey JOL: Anatomic aspects of vaginal eversion after hysterectomy, *Am J Obstet Gynecol* 166:1717–1724, 1992.

DeLancey JOL: Structural support of the urethra as it relates to stress urinary incontinence: the hammock hypothesis, *Am J Obstet Gynecol* 170:1713–1720, 1994.

DeLancey JOL: Structural anatomy of the posterior compartment as it relates to rectocele, *Am J Obstet Gynecol* 180:815–823, 1999.

Krantz KE: The anatomy of the urethra and anterior vaginal wall, *Am J Obstet Gynecol* 62:374–386, 1951.

Milley PS, Nichols DH: The relationship between the pubo-urethral ligaments and the urogenital diaphragm in the human female, *Anat Rec* 170:281–283, 1971.

Morley GW, DeLancey JOL: Sacrospinous ligament fixation for eversion of the vagina, *Am J Obstet Gynecol* 158:872–881, 1988.

Nichols DH, Randall CL: *Vaginal surgery*, ed 3, Baltimore, 1989, Williams & Wilkins.

Richardson AC, Lyon JB, Williams NL: A new look at pelvic relaxation, *Am J Obstet Gynecol* 126:568–573, 1976.

Weber AM, Walters MD: Anterior vaginal prolapse: review of anatomy and techniques of surgical repair, *Obstet Gynecol* 89:311–318, 1997.

Whiteside JL, Walters MD: Anatomy of the obturator region: relations to a trans-obturator sling, *Int Urogynecol J Pelvic Floor Dysfunct* 15:223–226, 2004.

Zacharin RF: *Pelvic floor anatomy and the surgery of pulsion enterocele*, New York, 1985, Springer-Verlag.

Preoperative Evaluation and Staging of Patients with Pelvic Organ Prolapse

Mickey Karram MD

 Video Clips online

3-1 Live Demonstrations of a Variety of Women with Advanced Prolapse

The decision to perform a surgical intervention on a patient with pelvic organ prolapse (POP) should be based on the degree of interference that the prolapse creates in the patient's daily life. This chapter discusses how to best take a history, perform a physical examination, and stage the prolapse appropriately. In addition, how to select the appropriate procedure to fit the patient's condition and how to guide patients through the preoperative consent process are also presented.

Taking a Good History

Patients with POP may report symptoms directly related to the prolapse, such as vaginal bulge, pressure, and discomfort, as well as a plethora of functional derangements related to voiding, defecation, and sexual problems.

Patients with POP should be questioned about all aspects of pelvic floor dysfunction. In the author's opinion, symptoms related to the lower urinary tract, the lower gastrointestinal tract, sexual function, and pelvic pain should be distinguished from those symptoms directly related to tissue protrusion or prolapse.

A variety of standardized questionaires (Burrows, 2004) can be used to assess fully the patient's perception of her pelvic floor symptomatology. Preferably, the patient completes these questionnaires before beginning the interview process. Although not always possible, these questionnaires allow the health care provider to appreciate the daily impact of these various problems. A voiding diary, which a patient maintains for 1 to 3 days, may also be helpful; as many of these patients have significant lower urinary tract dysfunction.

The ultimate goal of the history is to appreciate—from the patient's standpoint—which symptoms are the most bothersome and to determine whether the symptoms are related to the anatomic descent of her tissues. Ultimately, the surgeon needs to determine how anatomic correction of the prolapse will impact function.

Because the correlation between anatomic descent and functional derangement is somewhat unpredictable, patients need to be given realistic expectations regarding the impact of the surgical repair on their various symptoms. The role that these symptoms play in the continuum of the prolapse should be explained to the patient in a way that she can understand. Since many of these topics are extremely sensitive, questionnaires can significantly assist in the process of taking a history, especially when supplied to the patient before her visit. The answers to the various questions are used to guide the discussion and may permit the patient to share details that would otherwise be difficult to verbalize.

Appreciating any co-morbidities related to the patient's ability to tolerate pelvic reconstructive surgery is also important. The history of significant cardiac disease, myocardial infarction, and pulmonary disease are examples of conditions that need to be evaluated before considering a surgical procedure. Pulmonary embolism is a major risk factor in all types of pelvic surgery, especially in those patients who require prolonged dorsal lithotomy positioning. Before any surgery, the surgeon should recognize risk factors for embolism and use proper interventions during and after the surgical procedure.

Vaginal prolapse in any compartment—anterior, apical, or posterior—can cause vaginal fullness, pain, and/or a protruding mass. In a recent study by Tan and colleagues (2005), the feeling of "a bulge or that something is falling outside the vagina" had a positive predictive value of 81% for POP, and the lack of this symptom had a negative predictive value of 76% for predicting prolapse at or past the hymen. Not surprisingly, an increased degree of prolapse, especially beyond the hymen, is associated with increased pelvic discomfort and the visualization of a protrusion. The association of Pelvic Organ Prolapse Quantification (POPQ) measurements during the examination with three commonly related symptoms—urinary splinting, digital assistance with defecation, and vaginal bulge—is shown in Figure 3-1.

Urinary incontinence and voiding difficulties can occur in association with anterior and apical vaginal prolapse. However, women with advanced degrees of prolapse may not have overt symptoms of stress incontinence because the prolapse may cause a mechanical obstruction of the urethra, thereby preventing urinary leakage. Instead, these women may perform manual replacement of the prolapse to accomplish voiding. Patients who require digital assistance to void, in general, have more advanced degrees of prolapse. In addition to the difficulty voiding, other urinary symptoms, such as urgency, frequency, and urge incontinence, are found in women with prolapse.

POP, especially in the apical and posterior compartments, can be associated with defecatory dysfunction, such as the need for manual assistance with defecation and

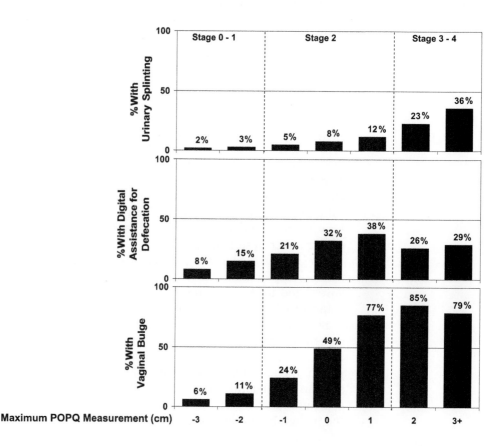

Figure 3-1 Prevalence of prolapse symptoms per the Pelvic Organ Prolapse Quantification (POPQ) system. The percentage of patients who report urinary splinting, digital assistance, and vaginal bulge is demonstrated for each relevant POPQ measurement.

(Modified from Tan JS, Lukacz ES, Menefee SA, et al: Predictive value of prolapse symptoms: a large database study, Int Urogynecol J Pelvic Floor Dysfunct *16:203-209, 2005.)*

anal incontinence of flatus, liquid, or solid stool. These patients often have outlet-type constipation, secondary to the trapping of stool within the rectocele, necessitating the need for splinting or for applying manual pressure in the vagina, rectum, or perineum to reduce the prolapse, which aids in defecation. Although defecatory dysfunction remains an area that is poorly understood in patients with prolapse, clinical and radiographic studies have shown that the severity of prolapse is not strongly correlated with increased symptoms.

Although the relationship between sexual function and POP is not clearly defined, questions regarding sexual dysfunction must be included in the evaluation of any patient with POP. Patients may report symptoms of dyspareunia and decreased libido and orgasms, as well as increased embarrassment because of an altered anatomy that affects body image. Some studies have reported that prolapse adversely affects sexual function, with subsequent improvement in sexual function after the repair of prolapse. (Barber et al, 2002; Rogers et al, 2001; Weber, Walters, Piedmonte, 2000) However, Burrows and associates (2004) showed little correlation between the extent of the prolapse and sexual dysfunction. Evaluating sexual function may be especially difficult in this patient population, secondary to the presence of factors other than prolapse, such as partner limitations and functional deficits.

Examination

When examining a patient with POP, a bimanual examination is performed to rule out co-existent gynecologic conditions.

The physical examination for prolapse should be conducted with the patient in the dorsal lithotomy position, as is used for a routine pelvic examination. If physical findings do not correspond to the reported symptoms or if the maximum extent of the prolapse cannot be confirmed, then the woman can be reexamined in the standing position. A rectal examination further identifies pelvic pathologic conditions and fecal impaction, the latter of which may be associated with voiding difficulties and incontinence in older women.

Initially, the external genitalia are inspected, and, if no displacement is apparent, the labia are gently spread to expose the vestibule and hymen. Vaginal discharge can mimic incontinence; therefore evidence of this problem should be sought and, if present, treated. Palpation of the anterior vaginal wall and urethra may elicit urethral discharge or tenderness that suggests a urethral diverticulum, carcinoma, or inflammatory condition of the urethra. The integrity of the perineal body is evaluated, and the extent of all prolapsed parts is assessed. A retractor, a Sims speculum, or the posterior blade of a bivalve speculum can be used to depress the posterior vagina to help visualize the anterior vagina and vice versa for the posterior vagina. The vaginal mucosa should be examined for atrophy and thinning, because both may affect the management of POP. Healthy, estrogenized tissue without significant evidence of prolapse will be well perfused, have rugation, and have physiologic moisture. Atrophic vaginal tissue consistent with hypoestrogenemia appears pale, thin, without rugation, and can be friable.

After the resting vaginal examination, the patient is instructed to perform a Valsalva maneuver or to cough vigorously. During this maneuver, the order and extent of the descent of the pelvic organs is noted, as is the relationship of the pelvic organs to each other at the peak of increased intraabdominal pressure. The presence and severity of anterior vaginal relaxation, including cystocele and proximal urethral detachment and mobility or anterior vaginal scarring, are estimated. Associated pelvic support abnormalities, such as rectocele, enterocele, and uterovaginal prolapse, are also noted. The amount or severity of prolapse in each vaginal segment should be measured and recorded using a standardized reproducible system for staging (see pages 34-37). A rectovaginal examination is required to evaluate fully the prolapse of the posterior vaginal wall and perineal body. Digital assessment of the bowel contents in the rectovaginal septum during the straining examination can help diagnose an enterocele. Inspection should also be made of the anal sphincter; as fecal incontinence can be associated with posterior vaginal support defects. Women with a torn external sphincter may have scarring or what has been termed a *dovetail sign*. **(See Video 3-1, "Live Demonstrations of a Variety of Women with Advanced Prolapse" 📹)**

Anterior vaginal wall descent usually represents bladder descent with or without concomitant urethral hypermobility. The anterior vaginal wall prolapse is believed to be the result of a midline defect, a paravaginal defect, or, less commonly, a transverse defect. These defects may co-exist or occur in isolation. Although clinicians have attempted to describe techniques to differentiate these various defects during the physical examination, researchers have shown that the preoperative predictability is not particularly reliable or accurate. In a study by Barber and associates (1999) of 117 women with prolapse, the sensitivity of the clinical examination to detect paravaginal defects (92%) was good, yet the specificity (52%) was poor. Despite a high prevalence of paravaginal defects, the positive predictive value was only 61%. Less than two thirds of women believed to have a paravaginal defect on physical examination were confirmed to possess the same at surgery. Another study by Whiteside and colleagues (2004) demonstrated poor predictability and reproducibility of the clinical examination to differentiate various anterior vaginal wall defects. Thus the clinical value of attempting to determine preoperatively the defect that is responsible for the anterior wall prolapse is low.

Clinical examinations do not always accurately differentiate rectoceles from enteroceles in posterior prolapse. Thus some investigators have advocated performing imaging studies to delineate further the exact nature of the posterior wall prolapse. Traditionally, most clinicians believe that they are able to detect the presence or absence of these defects without anatomically localizing them. However, little is known regarding the accuracy or use of clinical examinations in the evaluation of the anatomic locations of prolapsed small or large bowel or of specific defects in the rectovaginal space. Burrows and associates (2003) found that clinical examinations often did not accurately predict the specific location of defects in the rectovaginal septum that was subsequently found intraoperatively. Clinical findings corresponded with intraoperative observations in 59% of patients and differed in 41%; sensitivities and positive predictive values of clinical examinations were less than 40% for all posterior defects. However, the clinical consequence of not preoperatively detecting defects remains unclear.

Staging of Pelvic Organ Prolapse

The systemic descriptions and classifications of POP are useful to help document and communicate the severity of the problem and to standardize definitions to improve the quality of research. The Baden-Walker halfway system and the POPQ system are the two grading tools that are commonly used.

The Baden-Walker halfway system is a simple technique that is used to describe the severity of prolapse using criteria modified from Beecham (1980) and Baden and colleagues (1968). This grading system is simple to use and has reasonable interobserver variability for all segments of the vagina and for uterine support. The most dependent position of the pelvic organs during maximum straining or standing is used and graded as normal, first-, second-, and third-degree prolapse. First-degree prolapse is used for vaginal segments that descend halfway (but not to) the hymen; second-degree describes prolapse that descends to the hymen; and third-degree describes prolapse beyond the hymen (Figure 3-2).

Bump and associates (1996) described the International Continence Society (ICS) standardization of terminology of POP. In the POPQ system, the pelvic organ anatomy is described during the physical examination of the external genitalia and vaginal canal. This descriptive system contains a series of site-specific measurements of the woman's pelvic organ support. Prolapse in each segment is evaluated and measured, relative to the hymen. The anatomic position of the six defined points for measurement should be centimeters above (or proximal) to the hymen (negative number) or centimeters below (or distal) to the hymen (positive number) with the plane of the hymen defined

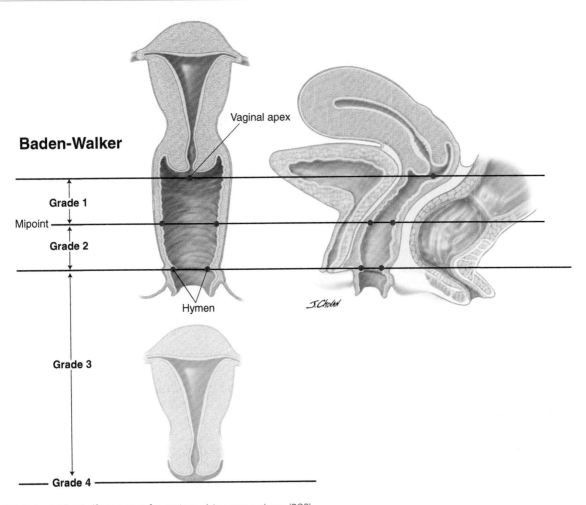

Figure 3-2 Baden-Walker halfway system for staging pelvic organ prolapse (POP).

(From Nitti VW, Rosenblum N, Brucker BM: Vaginal surgery for the urologist. In Karram M, editor: Female pelvic surgery video atlas series, *Philadelphia, 2012, Elsevier.)*

Figure 3-3 Pelvic Organ Prolapse Quantification (POPQ) system for staging pelvic organ prolapse (POP).

(From Nitti VW: Vaginal surgery for the urologist. In Karram M, editor: Female pelvic surgery video atlas series. *Philadelphia, 2012, Elsevier.)*

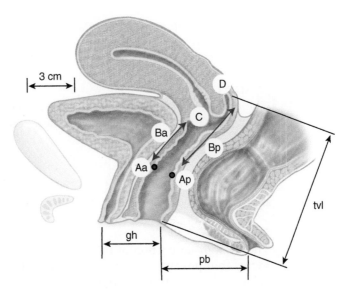

as zero. Six points are identified, which include two on the anterior vaginal wall, two in the superior vagina, and two on the posterior vaginal wall (Figure 3-3).

The two anterior sites are known and described as Point Aa and Point Ba. Points C and D are two points of the superior vagina and represent the most proximal locations of the normally positioned lower reproductive tract. Similar to the anterior vaginal wall are two points located on the posterior vaginal wall and are referred to as Point Bp and Point Ap. Specific definitions of these points include the following:

Point Aa: Located in the midline of the anterior vaginal wall, point Aa is 3 cm proximal to the external urethral meatus. By definition, the range of point Aa, relative to the hymen, is −3 to +3 cm.

Point Ba: Represents the most distal and most dependent point of any part of the upper anterior vaginal wall from the vaginal cuff or anterior vaginal fornix to point Aa. By definition, point Ba is at −3 in the absence of prolapse and would have a positive value equal to the position of the cuff in a woman with complete vaginal eversion.

Point C: Represents either the most distal edge of the cervix or the leading edge of the vaginal cuff after hysterectomy.

Point D: Measured only in women who have a cervix, point D represents a level of the uterosacral ligament attachment to the proximal posterior cervix and is included as a point of measurement to differentiate suspensory failure of the uterosacral cardinal ligament complex from cervical elongation.

Point Bp: Represents the most distal position of any part of the upper posterior vaginal wall from the vaginal cuff or posterior vaginal fornix to point Ap. By definition, point Bp is at −3 cm in the absence of prolapse and would have a positive value equal to the position of the cuff in a woman with post hysterectomy vaginal vault eversion.

Point Ap: Located in the midline of the posterior vaginal wall, point Ap is 3 cm proximal to the hymen. By definition, the range of position of point Ap, relative to the hymen, is −3 to +3 cm.

Other landmarks include the genital hiatus, which is measured from the middle of the external urethral meatus to the posterior midline of the hymen; and perineal body, which is measured from the posterior margin of the genital hiatus to the midanal opening. The total vaginal length is the greatest depth of the vagina in centimeters when point C or D is reduced to its full normal position.

The profile for quantifying prolapse provides a precise description of anatomy for individual patients. The five stages of pelvic organ support (0 to IV) are described in Box 3-1 and demonstrated in Figure 3-4. A grid and line diagram of a configuration can be drawn to organize and record measurements concisely (Figure 3-5).

Box 3-1 Stages of Pelvic Organ Prolapse

STAGE 0
No prolapse is demonstrated. Points Aa, Ap, Ba, and Bp are all at −3 cm, and either point C or D is between −TVL cm and −(TVL−2) cm; the quantitation value for point C or D is −(TVL−2) cm or less.

STAGE I
The criteria for stage 0 are not met, but the most distal portion of the prolapse is more than 1 cm above the level of the hymen; its quantitation value is less than −1 cm.

STAGE II
The most distal portion of the prolapse is from 1 cm proximal to 1 cm distal to the plane of the hymen; its quantitation value is −1, 0, or +1 cm.

STAGE III
The most distal portion of the prolapse is more than 1 cm below the plane of the hymen but protrudes no further than 2 cm less than the TVL; its quantitation value is more than +1 cm but less than +(TVL−2) cm.

STAGE IV
Essentially, complete eversion of the total length of the lower genital tract is demonstrated. The distal portion of the prolapse protrudes to at least TVL−2 cm; its quantitation value is +TVL−2 cm or more. In most instances, the leading edge of stage IV prolapse is the cervix or vaginal cuff scar.

TLV, Total vaginal length. From Bump RC, Mattiasson A, Bø K, et al: The standardization of terminology of female pelvic organ prolapse and pelvic floor dysfunction, Am J Obstet Gynecol 175:10–17, 1996.

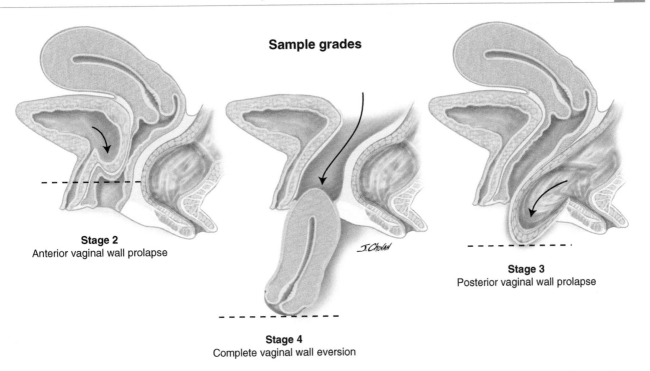

Sample grades

Stage 2
Anterior vaginal wall prolapse

J.Chovan

Stage 4
Complete vaginal wall eversion

Stage 3
Posterior vaginal wall prolapse

Figure 3-4 Stages 2, 3, and 4 of pelvic organ prolapse (POP) are illustrated. *(From Nitti VW: Vaginal surgery for the urologist. In Karram M, editor: Female pelvic surgery video atlas series, Philadelphia, 2012, Elsevier.)*

Ancillary techniques for describing POP include the following:

1. A digital rectal examination is performed while the patient is straining. This technique determines the extent of a rectocele and can also help corroborate the patient's complaint of splinting or having to manipulate her posterior vaginal wall or perineum to evacuate her bowels efficiently.

2. The contents of the rectovaginal septum are digitally assessed to differentiate a high rectocele from an enterocele.

3. A cotton swab test is performed to assess urethral mobility.

4. The perineal descent is measured.

5. The transverse diameter of the genital hiatus or the protruding prolapse is measured.

6. The extent of rectal prolapse, if present, is described and measured.

Evaluation of Bladder: Function

Commonly, patients with POP will also complain of lower urinary tract dysfunction. An office evaluation of voiding dysfunction in patients with prolapse should involve an assessment of voiding, detrusor function during filling, and competency of the urethral sphincteric mechanism. During the assessment of patients who complain of incontinence, the specific circumstances leading to the involuntary loss of urine should be determined. If possible, such circumstances should be reproduced and directly observed during clinical evaluation. The examination is most easily performed with the patient's bladder comfortably full. The patient is allowed to void as normally as possible in private. The time to void and the amount of urine voided is recorded. The patient then returns to the examination room, and the volume of residual urine is noted by transurethral catherization. If a sterile urine sample has not yet been obtained for analysis, it can be obtained at this time. A Toomey or Asepto syringe without its piston or bulb is attached to the catheter and held above the bladder. The patient is then asked

Figure 3-5 Diagram of pelvic organ prolapse (POP) created by recording measurements.

(From Nitti VW: Vaginal surgery for the urologist. In Karram M, editor: Female pelvic surgery video atlas series, *Philadelphia, 2012, Elsevier.)*

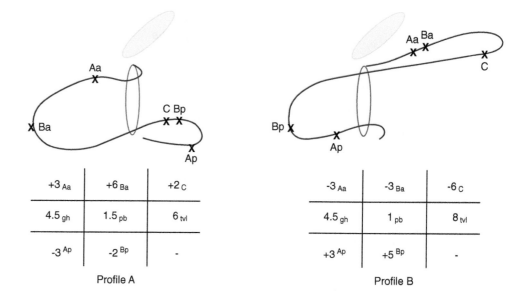

+3 Aa	+6 Ba	+2 C
4.5 gh	1.5 pb	6 tvl
-3 Ap	-2 Bp	-

Profile A

-3 Aa	-3 Ba	-6 C
4.5 gh	1 pb	8 tvl
+3 Ap	+5 Bp	-

Profile B

Figure 3-6 Office evaluation of bladder-filling function. In the sitting or standing position with a catheter in the bladder, the bladder is filled by gravity by pouring sterile water into the syringe.

(From Walters MD, Karram MM, editors: Urogynecology and reconstructive pelvic surgery, *ed 3, Philadelphia, 2007, Elsevier.)*

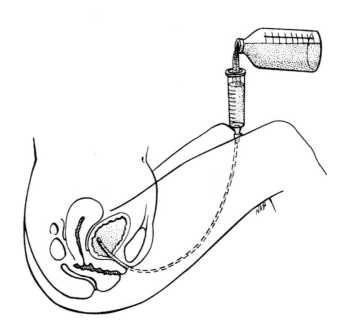

to sit or stand and the bladder is filled by gravity by pouring 50 ml aliquots of sterile water into the syringe (Figure 3-6). The patient's first bladder sensation and maximum bladder capacity are noted. The water level in the syringe should be closely observed during filling; any rise in the column of water can be secondary to a detrusor contraction and should be observed and recorded. Unintended increases in intraabdominal pressure by the patient should be avoided. The catheter is then removed, and the patient is asked to cough while in a supine position. If no leakage occurs and it appears that the prolapse is either kinking or obstructing the urethra, then a reduction maneuver should be performed to determine whether the patient has occult or potential stress incontinence. The goal of any reduction maneuver should be to duplicate the position of the vaginal tissue after a reconstructive procedure for prolapse. Overzealous reduction of tissue, in which a complete straightening of the posterior urethrovesical angle or aggressive downward traction with a speculum occurs (thus paralyzing the levator ani muscle), will falsely create stress incontinence in a large percentage of women. If no leakage is observed while the patient is in the supine position, the same maneuvers should be attempted with the patient in the standing position. A loss of small amounts of urine in spurts, simultaneous with the coughs, strongly suggests a diagnosis of urodynamic stress incontinence. Prolonged loss of urine, leaking a few seconds after coughing, or no urine loss with provocation may indicate other causes of incontinence, such as detrusor over activity. The interpretation of these office tests can be difficult because of the artifact introduced by rises in intraabdominal pressure caused by straining and patient movement. Borderline or negative tests should be repeated to maximize their diagnostic accuracy. This simple *eyeball* office filling study is a worthy screening test to perform before surgical intervention on all patients with prolapse. Formal urodynamics and cystoscopic testing should be considered in complicated or recurrent cases.

Laboratory Tests

Few laboratory tests are necessary for the evaluation of prolapse. A urine sample should be obtained for dipstick urinalysis. Urine culture and sensitivity tests should be obtained when the dipstick test indicates infection.

Acute cystitis can cause multiple irritative symptoms, such as dysuria, frequency, urgency, incontinence, and voiding difficulty. In these cases, treatment of the infection usually eradicates the symptoms. However, bacteriuria is often asymptomatic, especially in older women. Boscia and colleagues (1986) demonstrated that no differences in urinary symptoms were found in older patients with bacteriuria when compared with their nonbacteriuric state. In view of the conflicting data, examining the urine for infection in all patients who are incontinent seems reasonable; if bacteriuria is found, prescribing appropriate antibiotics and reevaluating the patient in several weeks are the treatments of choice.

Blood testing blood urea nitrogen (BUN), creatinine, glucose, and calcium levels is recommended if compromised renal function is suspected or if polyuria (in the absence of diuretics) is present. Urine cytologic testing is not recommended in the routine evaluation of the patient who is incontinent. However, patients with microscopic hematuria (two to five red blood cells per high power field), those older than 50 years of age with persistent hematuria, or those with acute onset of irritative voiding symptoms in the absence of urinary tract infection require cystoscopic imaging and cytologic testing to exclude bladder neoplasm.

Radiologic Assessment

After a careful history and physical examination, few diagnostic tests are needed to further evaluate patients with POP if no concomitant voiding or defecatory dysfunction is present. Although hydronephrosis occurs in a small percentage of women with prolapse, it usually does not change the management of the women for whom surgical repair is planned. Therefore routing imaging of the kidneys and ureters is not necessary.

As discussed earlier in this chapter, preoperative clinical assessment of specific support defects involved in prolapse often do not correspond to subsequent intraoperative findings. Therefore some investigators have advocated using imaging procedures such as ultrasonography, contrast radiography, and magnetic resonance imaging (MRI) to further describe the exact nature of the support defects before attempting surgical repairs. For example, some clinicians have used contrast ultrasonography to evaluate for paravaginal defects by placing a water-filled condom in the vaginal canal to delineate the paravaginal spaces. (Ostrzenski, Osborne, Ostrzenska, 1997) Others have used MRI to characterize more accurately the soft tissue and viscera of the pelvis. However, standardized radiologic criteria are currently lacking for diagnosing POP. Therefore the clinical use of imaging studies remains unknown and is currently used most often for research purposes.

Patients with prolapse who are without symptoms of defecatory dysfunction generally do not warrant ancillary bowel testing. For example, although defecating proctographic studies can provide additional information regarding rectal emptying, Siproudhis and colleagues (1993) demonstrated that this procedure is no more sensitive at detecting rectoceles than physical examination alone. However, patients with posterior vaginal wall prolapse and concomitant bowel dysfunction or mobility disorders merit further evaluation. In such a group of patients, differentiating between those with colonic motility disorders and those with pelvic outlet symptoms is important. Useful ancillary tests include anoscopic and proctosigmoidoscopic examination to evaluate for prolapsing hemorrhoids and intrarectal prolapse. Motility disorders can be assessed with colonic transit studies. In patients with apical and posterior vaginal prolapse who also complain of difficult or incomplete bowel emptying, evaluating for pelvic floor dyssynergia is important. During the physical examination, patients with pelvic floor dyssynergia often have hypercontracted and tender puborectalis muscles that may not relax on command. Tests for diagnosing pelvic floor dyssynergia include electromyography and a balloon expulsion test, which demonstrate a paradoxical contraction of the puborectalis muscle during defecation. Defecating proctography, which involves dynamic and still images of patients at rest during defecation and while contracting the anal sphincter, can also be used for diagnosis. Defecographic evaluation has the added advantage of providing radiographic evidence of the specific organ that is herniating into the posterior vaginal wall and is the "gold standard" for measuring perineal descent. This technique also shows how the contrast medium gets trapped in a rectocele that is creating the outlet obstruction.

Dynamic MRI defecography can also provide information regarding defecation and anatomic soft tissue defects. It has the advantages of being noninvasive, does not require ionizing radiation, and is unrivaled in its depictions of pelvic soft tissue. However, the clinical use of this costly imaging modality is debatable because it has not yet been shown to alter clinical decision making.

Selecting the Appropriate Procedure to Meet Patient Needs and to Complete the Consent Process

The goal of any procedure for POP should be to correct the anatomic descent in a durable fashion, as well as restore or maintain visceral and sexual function. Specific anatomic goals should be to reconstruct a vagina of adequate length (usually a minimum of 7 cm) with adequate vaginal caliber. Whatever surgical procedure is used to correct the POP, it should be individualized to meet these specific goals. Ultimately, the most important goal of the repair is to provide a durable high fixation of the vaginal vault in such a way that minimal deviation of the vaginal axis occurs. The vagina is extremely sensitive to its axis, and significant distortion of the vaginal axis commonly results in the development of prolapse in the segment of the vagina opposite the distortion; examples include the development of a posterior vaginal wall prolapse after colposuspension procedures and the development of an anterior vaginal wall prolapse after sacrospinous colpopexy. Ideally, the vaginal vault should sit on the levator plate, creating a slight posterior deviation of the upper vagina, which is what is accomplished when an abdominal sacral colpopexy is performed.

The upcoming chapters discuss a variety of procedures that can be used to correct POP. The various procedures are presented and described in the context of specific clinical case scenarios. The cases are then usually followed with a discussion of the reason the author of this text believes the specific procedure was chosen to meet the goals of the case presented.

Although providing a detailed discussion of the consent process is beyond the scope of this chapter, suffice it to say that patients should be presented with realistic expectations regarding the potential complications and outcomes of the procedure to be performed. In the author's opinion, general consent guidelines should be standardized, requiring a full understanding by the patient that the procedure is being performed to address a quality-of-life problem, with a full discussion regarding long-term outcomes and potential complications. Patients in whom graft material or prolapse mesh kits are being used require consent regarding the risks and benefits specific to the graft or kit being used.

Suggested Readings

Baden WF, Walker TA, Lindsey JH: The vaginal profile, *Tex Med* 64:56–58, 1968.

Barber MD, Cundiff GW, Weidner AC, et al: Accuracy of clinical assessment of paravaginal defects in women with anterior vaginal wall prolapse, *Am J Obstet Gynecol* 181:87–90, 1999.

Barber MD, Visco AG, Wyman JF, et al: Sexual function in women with urinary incontinence and pelvic organ prolapse, *Obstet Gynecol* 99:281–289, 2002.

Beecham CT: Classification of vaginal relaxation, *Am J Obstet Gynecol* 136:957–958, 1980.

Boscia JA, Kobasa WD, Abrutyn E, et al: Lack of association between bacteriuria and symptoms in the elderly, *Am J Med* 81:979–982, 1986.

Bump RC, Mattiasson A, Bø K, et al: The standardization of terminology of female pelvic organ prolapse and pelvic floor dysfunction, *Am J Obstet Gynecol* 175:10–17, 1996.

Burrows LJ, Sewell C, Leffler KS, et al: The accuracy of clinical evaluation of posterior vaginal wall defects, *Int Urogynecol J Pelvic Floor Dysfunct* 14:160–163, 2003.

Burrows LJ, Meyn LA, Walters MD, et al: Pelvic symptoms in women with pelvic organ prolapse, *Obstet Gynecol* 104:982–988, 2004.

Ostrzenski A, Osborne NG, Ostrzenska K: Method for diagnosing paravaginal defects using contrast ultrasonographic technique, *J Ultrasound Med* 16:673–677, 1997.

Rogers GR, Villarreal A, Kammerer-Doak D, et al: Sexual function in women with and without urinary incontinence and/or pelvic organ prolapse, *Int Urogynecol J Pelvic Floor Dysfunct* 12:361–365, 2001.

Siproudhis L, Robert A, Vilotte J, et al: How accurate is clinical examination in diagnosing and quantifying pelvirectal disorders? A prospective study in a group of 50 patients complaining of defecatory difficulties, *Dis Colon Rectum* 36:430–438, 1993.

Tan JS, Lukacz ES, Menefee SA, et al: Predictive value of prolapse symptoms: a large database study, *Int Urogynecol J Pelvic Floor Dysfunct* 16:203–209, 2005.

Weber AM, Walters MD, Piedmonte MR: Sexual function and vaginal anatomy in women before and after surgery for pelvic organ prolapse and urinary incontinence, *Am J Obstet Gynecol* 182:1610–1615, 2000.

Whiteside JL, Barber MD, Paraiso MF, et al: Clinical evaluation of anterior vaginal wall support defects: interexaminer and intraexaminer reliability, *Am J Obstet Gynecol* 191:100–104, 2004.

Techniques for Vaginal Hysterectomy and Vaginal Trachelectomy in Patients with Pelvic Organ Prolapse

4

Mickey Karram MD

 Video Clips online

4-1 Simple Vaginal Hysterectomy in a Patient with Mild Uterovaginal Prolapse

4-2 Morcellation Techniques in Patients with an Unsuspected Enlarged Uterus

4-3 Technique for Vaginal Oophorectomy

4-4 Electrosurgical Device–Assisted Vaginal Hysterectomy

4-5 Modified McCall Culdoplasty

4-6 Vaginal Hysterectomy in a Patient with an Elongated Cervix

4-7 Vaginal Trachelectomy

Hysterectomy is the second most frequent operation performed in the United States, followed only by cesarean section. Approximately 600,000 hysterectomies are performed annually in the United States, creating an economic burden of over 5 billion dollars. The rate of hysterectomy in the United States is among the highest in the developed world; approximately 23% of American women have undergone a hysterectomy.

Over the last four decades, a steady decline has occurred in the annual incidence of hysterectomy from a peak of approximately 10.4 per 1000 women in 1975, 6 per 1000 women in 1997, and approximately 5.4 per 1000 women in 2000 to 2004, according to national estimates. Between the years of 1997 and 2005, the hysterectomy rate in the United States has decreased approximately 1.9% per year. Increasing rates have been the highest in women 45 years and older.

The most common reason a woman undergoes hysterectomy is uterine leiomyoma, followed by excessive uterine bleeding. Pelvic organ prolapse accounts for approximately 15% to 18% of all hysterectomies performed in the United States. Historically, hysterectomy has almost always been indicated at the time of surgical correction when uterine prolapse is present. However, an increasing number of options are available for uterine preservation in women with uterovaginal prolapse (see Chapter 5). Uterine prolapse is not usually an isolated event and is often associated with other pelvic support defects. A hysterectomy alone is rarely an adequate treatment for prolapse; typically, associated surgical repairs are also necessary. Even in rare cases of isolated uterine prolapse, an enterocele repair or vaginal vault suspension of some type or both are almost always required. A hysterectomy is often unnecessary in patients with an isolated anterior or posterior vaginal wall prolapse or both and what appears to be a well-supported uterus. Hysterectomy as part of a procedure for pelvic organ prolapse can, at times, be extremely straightforward when a symmetric uterovaginal prolapse of a normal sized uterus is present. However, the hysterectomy can, at times, be challenging if an unexpected uterine enlargement, elongated cervix, or unexpected pathologic abnormality is present. This chapter focuses on the techniques used to perform vaginal hysterectomy in these various situations.

Preoperative Considerations in Patients Undergoing Hysterectomy

Pregnancy should always be ruled out in all reproductive-age women on the day of surgery. Attention to preoperative details such as prophylactic antibiotics and the prevention of venous thrombotic events are important to ensure a safe outcome. The most important perioperative management protocols involve the use of timing the prophylactic antibiotics to decrease the risk of surgical site infection and treatments or maneuvers to prevent venous thrombotic events. A recent normal Papanicolaou test (Pap smear) should be documented before performing a hysterectomy. Sampling of the endometrium or pelvic ultrasound should also be considered in patients who are at risk for a malignancy such as women with postmenopausal bleeding and polycystic ovaries syndrome. Based on age alone, it is generally recommended that women older than 39 years of age with persistent and ovulatory bleeding have an endometrial assessment after excluding pregnancy. Some guidelines suggest a cut-off age of 35 years (American Congress of Obstetricians and Gynecologists [ACOG] Practice Bulletin No. 14, 2001). If a pelvic mass is palpated during the pelvic examination, a transvaginal ultrasound examination should be performed. No other imaging modality has been shown to be superior (ACOG Practice Bulletin No. 83, 2007). If a suspicious mass is found on a transvaginal ultrasound examination, then appropriate consultation with a gynecologic oncologist is recommended before surgery. Uterine prolapse is often accompanied by other pelvic floor disorders, including bladder and bowel dysfunction. These problems also need to be evaluated preoperatively and addressed surgically if appropriate at the time of hysterectomy.

Informed consent for hysterectomy should be a process rather than a single event. Multiple factors need to be documented, including whether the patient has completed childbearing. The patient should always be warned that the potential exists for the conversion of the hysterectomy to a laparoscopic and or abdominal route if complications occur that cannot be transvaginally addressed. (For a broader discussion on hysterectomy, the reader is referred to Walters M, Barber M, editors: Hysterectomy for benign disease. In Karram M, editor: *Female pelvic surgery video atlas series,* Philadelphia, 2010, Elsevier.)

Case 1: Vaginal Hysterectomy and McCall Culdoplasty for Mild Uterovaginal Prolapse

 View: Video 4-1

A 43-year-old woman (gravida 3, para 2) complains of mildly symptomatic pelvic organ prolapse and dysfunctional uterine bleeding. She has previously undergone an endometrial ablation that controlled her abnormal bleeding for approximately 1 year. Over the past 9 months, however, she has experienced significantly more bleeding and is changing pads on a regular basis. Her menses are also associated with significant cramping and some low back pain. During the physical examination, a cystocele is noted in which the anterior vaginal wall descends to the hymen when she strains in a supine position (Points Aa and Ba are at zero). The cervix descends to approximately 2 centimeters within the hymen (Point C is −2 cm), and she has relatively good support of the posterior vaginal wall. She also admits to some mild stress incontinence, which is confirmed on urodynamic testing. She desires definitive therapy; after a detailed discussion of the risks and benefits, the decision is made to perform a vaginal hysterectomy with a McCall culdoplasty and a suture repair of the anterior and possibly the posterior vaginal walls, as well as a synthetic midurethral sling for her stress incontinence.

Procedural Details

1. Before surgery, perioperative intravenous antibiotics and antiembolic prophylaxis are routinely administered.

2. Appropriate positioning of a patient for vaginal hysterectomy includes the patient being in dorsal lithotomy position with her feet in candy cane or Allen stirrups. The patient's buttocks extend slightly over the table so that the posterior retractor can be easily placed. The thighs are somewhat abducted and the hips are flexed. Excessive flexion and abduction of the thigh are avoided, which can lead to position-induced injuries. Candy cane stirrups are preferred for deep vaginal surgery and when two vaginal surgical assistants are needed.

3. Examination under anesthesia is performed to confirm the uterine size, the degree of uterine mobility, the width of the vaginal canal, and the presence or absence of pelvic pathologic abnormalities. The freedom of the cul de sac is noted, and a rectovaginal bimanual examination is performed.

4. The vaginal, perineal, and lower abdominal areas are prepared in normal fashion, and the patient is sterilely draped. The urinary bladder is then emptied by a catheter, or an indwelling Foley catheter is placed for continual drainage.

5. The cervix is grasped with two single-tooth uterine tenacula, and downward traction is placed. The author prefers to use a vasoconstrictor agent such as vasopressin or a prepared solution of 0.5 % lidocaine; 1:200,000 epinephrine can be used if no contraindications exist. The solution is injected into the cervix or paracervical tissue just before the incision is made, which has been shown to decrease operative blood loss without an increase in morbidity in randomized trials. The maximum amount of lidocaine administered with epinephrine should not exceed 7 mg/kg body weight or 500 mg total in a healthy adult. Should a medical contraindication be present to the use of vasopressors or epinephrine, injectable saline provides the benefits of hydrodistention without the benefit of vasoconstriction or any increase in cardiovascular risk.

6. A knife or electrosurgical instrument is used to make the initial incision through the vaginal mucosa at the cervicovaginal junction (Figure 4-1). The position and depth of this incision is extremely important, and, if performed correctly, significantly facilitates the simplicity of the hysterectomy. The appropriate location of this incision is at the site of the bladder reflection, which is identified by a crease formed in the vaginal mucosa when the cervix is pushed slightly inward. If the location cannot be identified, the incision is made lower rather than higher to avoid any potential bladder injury. The circumferential incision is cut down until the cervical stroma is encountered. A clear plane exists between the full thickness of the vaginal wall and the cervical stroma. When this plane is reached, the vaginal tissue falls away from the underlying cervical tissue; this direct plane leads the surgeon to both the anterior and posterior cul-de-sacs.

7. Posterior mobilization of the vagina allows access to the posterior cul-de-sac, which is sharply entered with Mayo scissors and then explored digitally for any adhesive diseases, masses, or bowel, as well as to confirm the size of the uterus (Figures 4-2 and 4-3).

8. Downward traction on the uterus and pulling it to one side facilitates the placement of the first clamp. A Heaney or Ballentine clamp is used to ligate the uterosacral ligament (Figure 4-4). This pedicle is cut with Mayo scissors and ligated with an absorbable suture. The authors prefer an O-vicryl suture on a CT1 needle. The cut pedicle is suture ligated with a type of transfixing suture in which the needle enters the upper part of the ligament pedicle just behind the tip of the Heaney clamp; it is withdrawn and then reintroduced into the pedicle at its midpoint. This suture has been termed a *Heaney-type stitch*. Each uterosacral ligament is usually tagged for later identification.

9. Sharp dissection is then used to further mobilize the vaginal wall off the cervix, and the cardinal ligaments are bilaterally clamped and ligated in a similar fashion. Careful and concise incisions are used to enter the anterior cul-de-sac to prevent any inadvertent cystotomy (Figure 4-5). In addition, forceful blunt dissection of the bladder off the cervix with a finger or a sponge stick is discouraged because lacerations can occur. Many women who have had previous

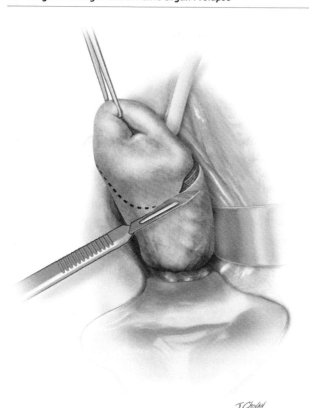

Figure 4-1 A scalpel is used to make the initial incision through the vaginal mucosa at the cervicovaginal junction.

(From Walters MD, Barber MD: Hysterectomy for benign disease. In Karram M, editor: Female pelvic surgery video atlas series, Philadelphia, 2010, Elsevier.)

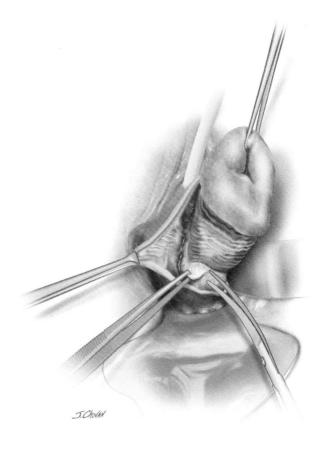

Figure 4-2 After the vagina is dissected from the cervix, the posterior cul-de-sac is sharply entered with Mayo scissors.

(From Walters MD, Barber MD: Hysterectomy for benign disease. In Karram M, editor: Female pelvic surgery video atlas series, Philadelphia, 2010, Elsevier.)

cesarean sections may exhibit significant scarring between the anterior vaginal wall and the base of the bladder. No attempt to enter the anterior cul-de-sac is made until the vesicouterine space has been developed and the preperitoneal tissue has been visualized (Figure 4-6). Once the vesicouterine space has been entered, a retractor is used to elevate the bladder off the uterus, and the anterior cul-de-sac peritoneum can be entered. A Heaney retractor is then placed anteriorly using a finger to protect the bladder (Figure 4-7).

10. The next clamp usually includes the uterine vessels and incorporates anterior and posterior peritoneal reflections of both cul-de-sacs. The placement of these clamps is perpendicular to the longitudinal axis of the cervix, and the tips of the clamps slide off the tip of the cervix and uterus to ensure that all of the parametrical and vascular tissues have been included (Figure 4-8). This placement of the clamps helps avoid excessive bleeding and clearly ensures that the surgeon is staying close to the cervix, which should avoid any potential for ureteral injury. The uterine vessels are then suture ligated with a fixation stitch in which each pedicle is sutured into the previous pedicle. This technique completely obliterates the dead space between pedicles, thus decreasing the potential for the tearing of tissue and bleeding (Figure 4-9). Depending on the size of the uterus, several more clamps may be needed. If the uterus is enlarged, then morcellation techniques are used and usually started at this point. **(See Video 4-2, "Morcellation Techniques in Patients with an Unsuspected Enlarged Uterus."**)
Once the adnexal pedicles have been identified, the uterus can usually be posteriorly delivered through the vagina by grasping the fundus with a tenaculum and pulling downward to expose the uterovaginal ligament. A Heaney clamp is placed close to the uterus, clamping the pedicles. Usually, one clamp is sufficient; however, at times, two clamps may be needed if the pedicle is

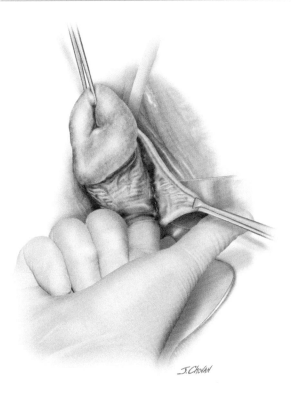

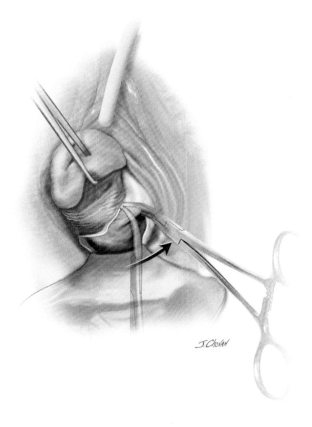

Figure 4-3 After sharp entry into the posterior cul-de-sac, the peritoneal cavity is digitally explored for any adhesive disease, masses, or bowel, as well as to confirm that damage to the rectum has not occurred.

(From Walters MD, Barber MD: Hysterectomy for benign disease. In Karram M, editor: Female pelvic surgery video atlas series, *Philadelphia, 2010, Elsevier.)*

Figure 4-4 The Heaney clamp is introduced into the posterior cul-de-sac and rotated toward the horizontal position; the uterosacral ligament is then clamped.

(Modified from Walters MD, Barber MD: Hysterectomy for benign disease. In Karram M, editor: Female pelvic surgery video atlas series, *Philadelphia, 2010, Elsevier.)*

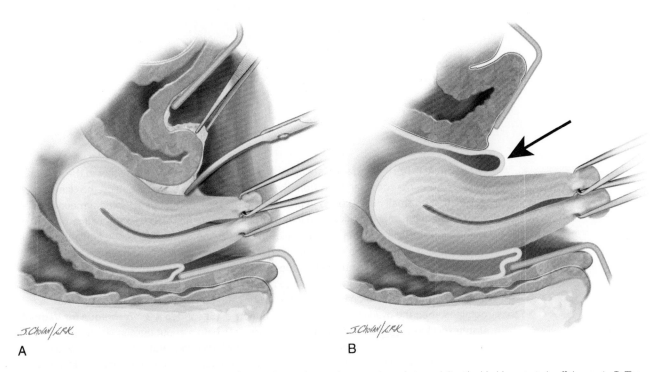

A   B

Figure 4-5 A, Sharp dissection with Mayo or Metzenbaum scissors close to the uterus is made to mobilize the bladder anteriorly off the cervix. **B,** The bladder is dissected off the uterus until the lower edge of the peritoneum is visualized *(arrow).*

(From Walters MD, Barber MD: Hysterectomy for benign disease. In Karram M, editor: Female pelvic surgery video atlas series, *Philadelphia, 2010, Elsevier.)*

Figure 4-6 Adhesions between the bladder and cervix from a previous cesarean section are noted. These are best taken down with sharp dissection **(A)**. Blunt dissection may lead to an inadvertent cystotomy, because the finger will pass into the area of least resistance **(B)**.

(From Walters MD, Barber MD: Hysterectomy for benign disease. In Karram M, editor: Female pelvic surgery video atlas series, *Philadelphia, 2010, Elsevier.)*

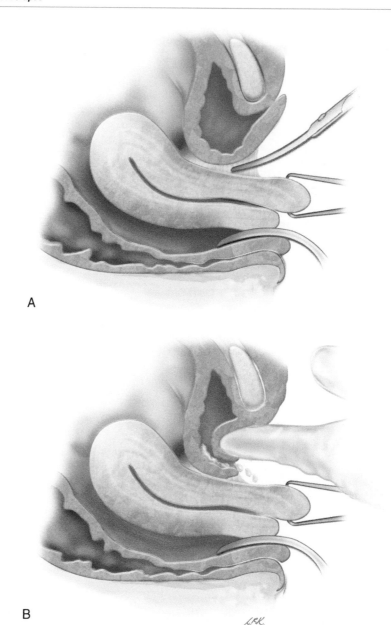

A

B

large (Figure 4-10). If two clamps are used, then they should overlap each other in the midline. Before cutting the specimen away from the clamps, the finger is placed behind the clamps to ensure that no small bowel comes in proximity to the back of the uterus. Some surgeons prefer double ligating this pedicle first with a free suture and then followed by a suture ligature. Once both clamps have incised the specimen (i.e., the uterus and cervix), it is handed off and sent for a pathologic evaluation. The clamps are then retracted and the adnexal structures (i.e., ovaries and tubes) are palpated to ensure that they are normal and that no unsuspecting pathologic abnormalities exist. If the adnexa are to be removed following the preference of the patient or if an abnormality or a lesion is found in the ovaries and patient consent has been previously obtained, then the ovaries and tubes can be removed. **(See Video 4-3, "Technique for Vaginal Oophorectomy."**) The ovarian ligature sutures are held without tension, as are the uterosacral pedicles. (For a detailed discussion on the indications and techniques for vaginal oophorectomy at the time of vaginal hysterectomy, the reader is referred to Walters M, Barber M; editors: Hysterectomy for benign disease. In Karram M, editor: *Female pelvic surgery video atlas series,* Philadelphia, 2010, Elsevier.)

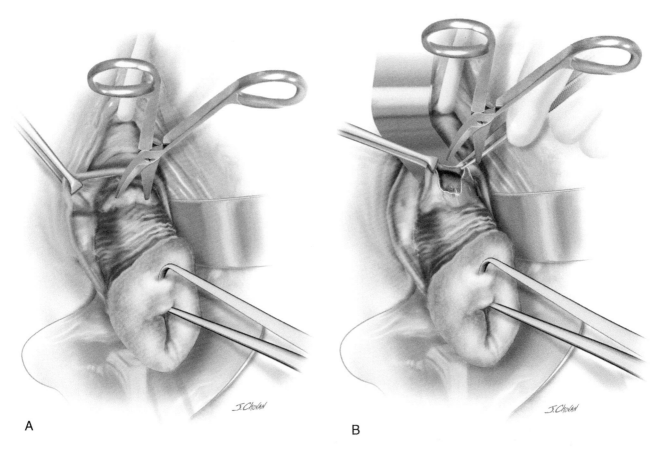

A   B

Figure 4-7 A, The anterior peritoneum is carefully inspected and palpated to differentiate it from the bladder. **B,** The anterior peritoneum is incised with scissors.

(From Walters MD, Barber MD: Hysterectomy for benign disease. In Karram M, editor: Female pelvic surgery video atlas series, *Philadelphia, 2010, Elsevier.)*

11. Some surgeons prefer an electrosurgical bypass or vessel-sealing device to seal or fuse the blood vessels instead of using the traditional methods of clamping, cutting, and suture-ligating these pedicles. The tissue effusion instrument consists of a disposable device with a pistol grip, Heaney-type clamp, and retractable scalpel to cut tissue after fusion. Pedicles are clamped, sealed, and fused; they are then cut before the clamp is released. This device is then advanced to the next pedicle, and the process is repeated. Although no randomized trials have compared this procedure with the traditional clamping techniques to verify clinical benefit, this technology is popular and has been shown in several small studies to decrease operating and anesthesia time, as well as patient blood loss. **(See Video 4-4, "Electrosurgical Device–Assisted Vaginal Hysterectomy."** 🎦**)**

12. At this time, the support of the vaginal cuff is assessed and the surgeon must determine whether a simple culdoplasty is sufficient to facilitate apical vaginal length or whether a formal apical suspension is needed. The author of this text believes that if the vaginal cuff descends to less than a −2 station after the uterus has been removed, then a McCall culdoplasty is an excellent mechanism to obliterate the enterocele, support the cuff to the uterosacral ligaments, and add sufficient posterior vaginal wall length. A McCall culdoplasty should almost routinely be considered in all vaginal hysterectomies whether performed for prolapse conditions or other gynecologic indications. In a randomized surgical trial, adding this maneuver, compared with simple vaginal closure, was shown to lower the risk of future prolapse. (Cruikshank, Kovac, 1999) The McCall culdoplasty is performed by passing nonabsorbable sutures from the vaginal lumen just lateral to the midline of the posterior vaginal wall into the peritoneal cavity. This same suture is then taken through the left uterosacral ligament across the intervening peritoneum and through the right uterosacral ligament; it then exits the vaginal cuff just to the

Figure 4-8 A, The uterine vessels are clamped with a Heaney clamp, incorporating posterior and anterior peritoneum, if possible. The handle of the clamp is rotated to nearly a horizontal position to facilitate suture placement. **B,** The uterine vessels are cut and sutured.

(Modified from Walters MD, Barber MD: Hysterectomy for benign disease. In Karram M, editor: Female pelvic surgery video atlas series, *Philadelphia, 2010, Elsevier.)*

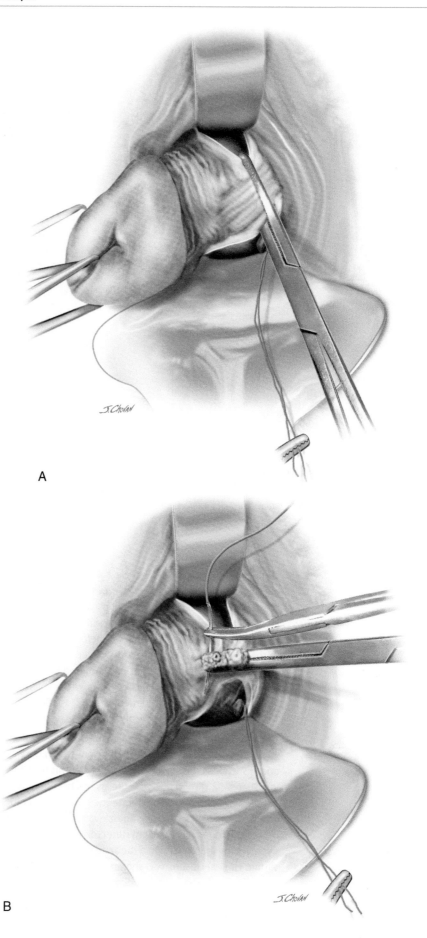

A

B

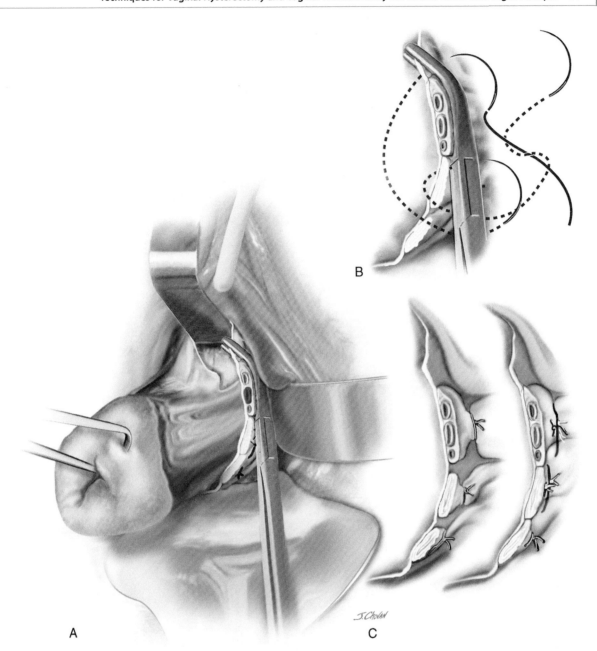

Figure 4-9 A, Proper technique for the clamping of the uterine vessels is demonstrated. **B,** The pedicle is sutured to ligate the vessels and to incorporate the pedicle into the previously ligated pedicle. A suture is initially passed through the tissue at the tip of the clamp; then a second pass of the needle is made through the distal end of the previous pedicle. **C,** The technique of completely ligating pedicles obliterates the dead space between pedicles. This technique is contrasted with the technique of individually ligating each pedicle, which results in gaps between pedicles that may lead to a tearing of tissue with bleeding between the pedicles.

(Modified from Baggish MS, Karram MM: Atlas of pelvic anatomy and gynecologic surgery, ed 3, St Louis, 2011, Elsevier.)

left of the midline. Numerous external sutures can be placed as needed. Internal McCall sutures, which are sutures that simply plicate the two uterosacral ligaments and intervening peritoneum, can then be placed as needed. External McCall sutures are always delayed absorbable sutures; as the knots are tied in the lumen of the vagina, while internal McCall sutures are permanent sutures because the knot is tied intraperitoneally (Figure 4-11). **(Video 4-5, "Modified McCall Culdoplasty," demonstrates the use of the McCall procedure** 🔊**).** A modification of the McCall culdoplasty, which is commonly used in patients with prolapse, involves the technique of removing a redundant wedge of the posterior vaginal wall and peritoneum (Figure 4-12).

Figure 4-10 The uterus is delivered through the posterior cul-de-sac, and the fallopian tube and the ovarian ligaments are clamped close to the uterus before cutting. To prevent accidental cutting of the bowel or other structures, a finger is behind the pedicle.

(From Walters MD, Barber MD: Hysterectomy for benign disease. In Karram M, editor: Female pelvic surgery video atlas series, Philadelphia, 2010, Elsevier.)

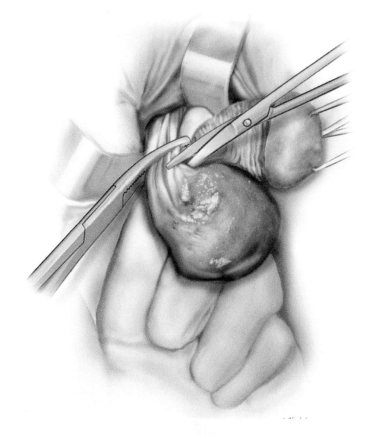

Figure 4-11 Proper suture placement of internal and external McCall stitches is demonstrated.

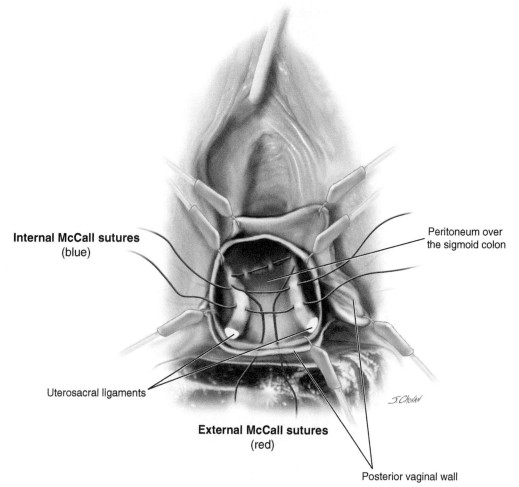

Internal McCall sutures (blue)

Peritoneum over the sigmoid colon

Uterosacral ligaments

External McCall sutures (red)

Posterior vaginal wall

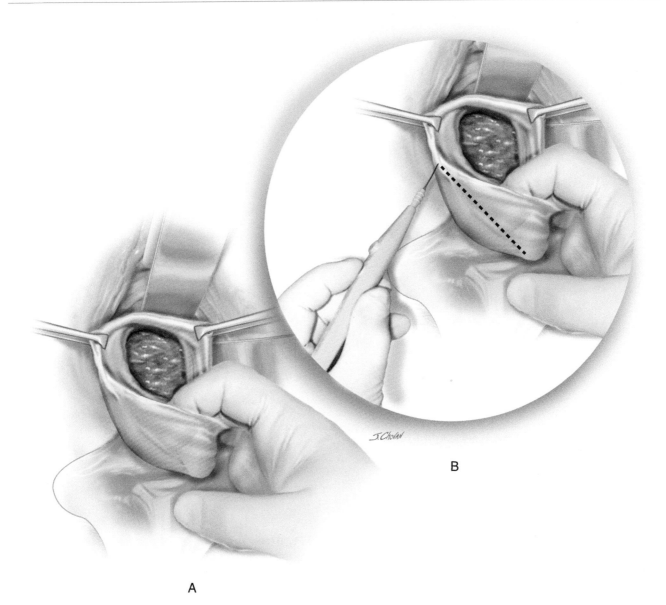

Figure 4-12 Digital palpation of the posterior cul-de-sac and enterocele is visualized. The technique of removal of the redundant wedge of the posterior vaginal wall and peritoneum are demonstrated *(inset)*.

(Modified from Baggish MS, Karram MM: Atlas of pelvic anatomy and gynecologic surgery, ed 3, St Louis, 2011, Elsevier.)

Case 2: Vaginal Hysterectomy for Advanced Uterovaginal Prolapse

A 72-year-old woman with a long-standing history of advanced uterovaginal prolapse complains of a protruding mass from the vagina, and she has recently developed significant lower urinary tract dysfunction (i.e., difficulty evacuating her bladder). The patient has to reduce the bulge manually to initiate her voids. She also admits to worsening urinary frequency, both diurnal and nocturnal, and describes the feeling of an incomplete bladder. A physical examination reveals that she has complete uterovaginal prolapse (stage IV) with a complete eversion of the anterior and posterior vaginal walls. The cervix protrudes approximately 8 cm beyond the hymen (Figure 4-13). She desires surgical correction of her prolapse and, after detailed discussion, understands that this corrective procedure involves a vaginal hysterectomy and appropriate suture repairs of her anterior and posterior vaginal walls with a vaginal vault suspension either to the uterosacral ligaments or the sacrospinous ligament.

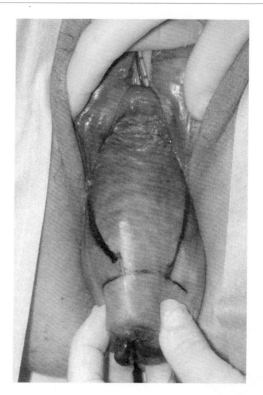

Figure 4-13 Uterovaginal prolapse. The displaced location of the bladder and ureters are demonstrated. The distal bladder reflection is marked by a horizontal line that is 2 to 3 cm above the anterior cervix. Ureteral catheters have been bilaterally placed, which allows the palpation of the distal ureter course that is also marked. The ureteral orifices are located just above the distal bladder reflection.

(Courtesy of W. Allen Addison, MD. Duke University Medical Center.)

Surgical Techniques Specific for Advanced Uterovaginal Prolapse

On preoperative examination, it is extremely important that the surgeon fully characterize the support of the anterior and posterior vaginal walls and the uterus, which will determine the symmetry (or lack thereof) of the prolapse as appropriate planning of the surgical repairs are made. In addition, the surgeon carefully palpates the cervix and uterus to determine whether cervical elongation is present, which is not an uncommon finding in patients with uterine prolapse. Assuming that the cervix is not elongated, the basic steps for hysterectomy in a patient with complete prolapse are similar to those of the standard vaginal hysterectomy previously described. The principal surgical challenge in these patients is the distortion of the normal anatomic relationships. In the absence of cervical elongation, the distal reflection of the bladder is 2 to 3 cm proximal to the cervix; therefore the initial vaginal dissection should be made just proximal to the distal cervix. Eversion of the bladder trigone displaces the ureteral orifices distally (see Figure 4-13). Thus significantly altering the course of the distal ureters. The surgeon dissects close to the cervix and protects the bladder with retractors throughout the procedure. Typically, the posterior cul-de-sac, which may contain prolapsing small intestine (i.e., enterocele), lies behind the upper half of the posterior vaginal wall; the distal rectum lies behind the distal posterior vaginal wall. Usually, entry into the posterior cul-de-sac during hysterectomy for advanced uterovaginal prolapse is easily accomplished, but an anterior entry can be more challenging. Once posterior entry occurs and if the uterus is small, then a finger can be usually passed through the posterior cul-de-sac around the uterus to tent up the anterior peritoneum and to aid in anterior entry. The remaining steps are identical to that for a vaginal hysterectomy. Usually, postmenopausal patients have small uteruses; therefore two or three clamps on each side are all that are necessary before delivering the uterus through the vaginal incision. Once the hysterectomy is completed, an extensive vaginal reconstructive procedure is always necessary to address the other aspects of the prolapse, specifically the anterior and posterior vaginal walls and, most importantly, the vaginal apex. (See chapters 7-9 for more details regarding these portions of the procedure.)

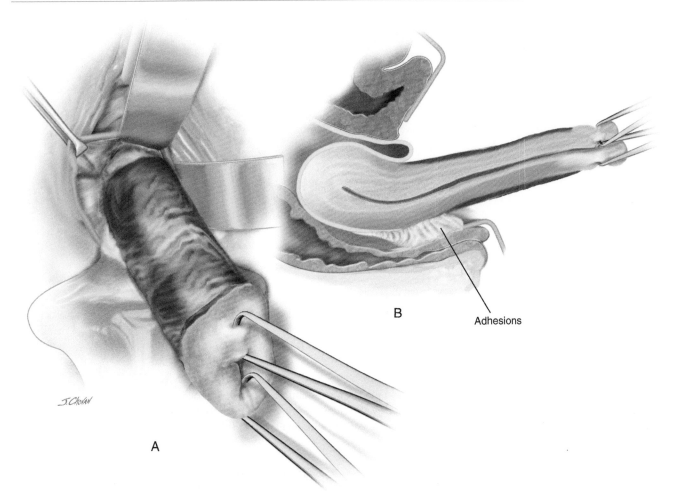

Figure 4-14 A, A significantly elongated cervix with a high anterior cul-de-sac is visualized. Usually, the reason a cervix is elongated is not obvious. **B,** However, as demonstrated in this figure, at times elongation may be a result of adhesive disease in the posterior or anterior cul-de-sac.

(Modified from Baggish MS, Karram MM: Atlas of pelvic anatomy and gynecologic surgery, *ed 3, St Louis, 2011, Elsevier.)*

In some patients with uterine prolapse, the cervix is significantly elongated, which is usually apparent during examination as the cervix is palpated. The cause of cervical elongation is largely unknown; however, it is more common in postmenopausal women. It can occur in isolation, in which the actual body of the uterus is well supported; however, it is often associated with varying degrees of uterovaginal prolapse. It occurs more frequently when the uterus is fixed and immobile from previous adhesive disease or previous uterine fixation. On preoperative examination, cervical elongation is often characterized by the cervix extending well into the vagina, and, in some patients, beyond the introitus (also called the *pseudoprolapse*). Typically, the posterior vaginal fornix is well supported with the fundus in a normal position within the pelvis, which differentiates it from true uterine prolapse (Figures 4-14 and 4-15). In patients with cervical elongation, the primary challenges include entry into the anterior and posterior cul-de-sacs because the peritoneal folds are much higher than usual. Before initiating the hysterectomy, simple palpation while the patient in under anesthesia usually reveals the location of the transition between the cervix and the fundus at the lower uterine segment. Rectal examination determines the distal extent of the rectum. Identifying the distal extent of the bladder is, at times, useful to help determine where to make the initial incision in the anterior vaginal wall. After identifying these landmarks, the surgeon can distally make the initial circumferential vaginal incision distal enough to avoid visceral injury and maintain appropriate vaginal length but also high enough to avoid unnecessary dissection on the distal aspect of the elongated cervix. In patients with cervical elongation, performing extensive dissection and potentially sequential suture ligation extraperitoneally for several bytes is almost always necessary before the anterior and posterior peritoneal folds are encountered (Figures 4-16 and 4-17). Once the anterior and posterior cul-de-sacs are entered, the remainder of the

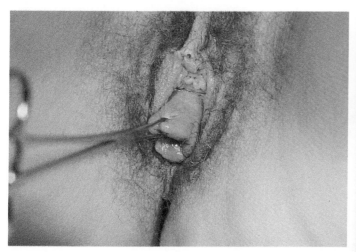

Figure 4-15 Uterine prolapse with a significantly elongated cervix.

(From Baggish MS, Karram MM: Atlas of pelvic anatomy and gynecologic surgery, *ed 3, St Louis, 2011, Elsevier.)*

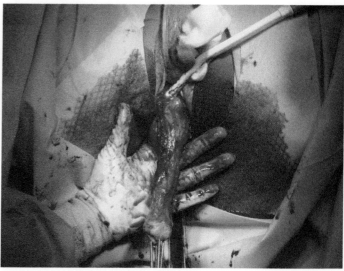

Figure 4-16 A significantly elongated cervix is demonstrated. Sharp dissection of the bladder off the anterior cervical wall is observed at the level of the vesicouterine space.

(From Baggish MS, Karram MM: Atlas of pelvic anatomy and gynecologic surgery, *ed 3, St Louis, 2011, Elsevier.)*

hysterectomy proceeds in the routine fashion. To gain more mobility or exposure during the remainder the hysterectomy, the elongated cervix can be amputated if necessary. **(See Video 4-6, "Vaginal Hysterectomy in a Patient with an Elongated Cervix."**)

Case 3: Vaginal Trachelectomy for Cervical Stump Prolapse

A 43-year-old patient (para 3) complains of a firm structure protruding outside the introitus at the end of the day and with coughing or straining. One year before presentation, she underwent a robotic supracervical hysterectomy for abnormal uterine bleeding. She has obvious cervical stump prolapse; the cervix descends 2 cm outside the hymen with straining in a supine position. She also has some associated anterior and posterior vaginal wall prolapse (Point Aa and Ba are at 0 station, and point Bp is at 0 station). She denies any lower urinary tract or bowel dysfunction. She desires definitive therapy and provides the consent for a vaginal trachelectomy with native tissue suture repair of the anterior and posterior vaginal walls, as well as a vaginal vault suspension to either the uterosacral ligaments for the sacrospinous ligaments.

Techniques for Vaginal Trachelectomy

The cervical stump is removed in an identical fashion to the initial steps of a vaginal hysterectomy. Although entering the peritoneal cavity is not mandatory, this entry is preferred to ensure the complete removal of the cervix and to allow for a culdoplasty or vaginal vault suspension, based on the extent of the prolapse. Figure 4-18 demonstrates how clamps are passed above the upper margin of the cervix after the bladder has been superiorly mobilized. The specimen is cut away, and the remainder of the procedure is performed in a fashion identical to a vaginal hysterectomy. **(See Video 4-7, "Vaginal Trachelectomy."**)

Discussion of the Case

A cervical stump is the remnant of the uterus that remains after a subtotal hysterectomy. Historically, supracervical hysterectomy is only performed under adverse circumstances whereby rapid termination of the procedure was essential for the well-being of the patient (e.g., in situations involving a complicated pregnancy). However, more recently, surgeons are electively performing laparoscopic or robotic subtotal hysterectomy. Subsequent removal of the stump or trachelectomy may be required for various reasons, including persistent bleeding, prolapse (as with this patient), pain, and cervical pathologic abnormalities.

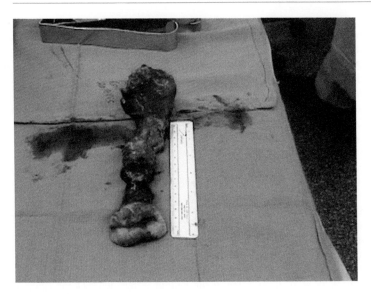

Figure 4-17 A significantly elongated cervix is visualized in a patient with uterine procidentia.

(Modified from Baggish MS, Karram MM: Atlas of pelvic anatomy and gynecologic surgery, ed 3, St Louis, 2011, Elsevier.)

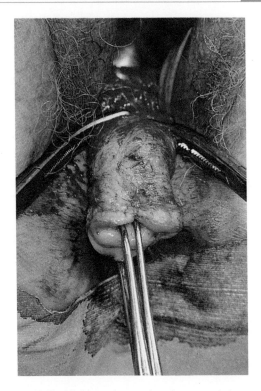

Figure 4-18 The bladder and ureters have been superiorly mobilized and out of the way of the clamps.

(From Baggish MS, Karram MM: Atlas of pelvic anatomy and gynecologic surgery, ed 3, St Louis, 2011, Elsevier.)

SUMMARY: In summary, uterovaginal hysterectomy for pelvic organ prolapse is still commonly performed, although uterine-preserving procedures have recently gained popularity. A detailed discussion of the long-term risks and benefits of vaginal hysterectomy versus uterine preservation needs to be undertaken with every patient with pelvic organ prolapse in which significant uterovaginal prolapse is presented. (For a more detailed discussion regarding the benefits of uterine preservation, the reader is referred to Chapter 5).

Suggested Readings

ACOG Practice Bulletin No. 14: Management of anovulatory bleeding. The American Congress of Obstetricians and Gynecologists, *Int J Gynaecol Obstet* 72:263–271, 2001.

ACOG Practice Bulletin No. 83: Management of adnexal masses. The American Congress of Obstetricians and Gynecologists, *Obstet Gynecol* 110:201–214, 2007.

ACOG Practice Bulletin No. 84: Prevention of deep vein thrombosis and pulmonary embolism. Committee on Practice Bulletins—Gynecology, the American Congress of Obstetricians and Gynecologists, *Obstet Gynecol* 110:429–440, 2007.

ACOG Practice Bulletin No. 89: Elective and risk-reducing salpingo-oophorectomy, *Obstet Gynecol* 111:231–241, 2008.

ACOG Committee Opinion No. 395: Surgery and patient choice. The American Congress of Obstetricians and Gynecologists, *Obstet Gynecol* 111:243–247, 2008.

Ascher-Walsh CJ, Capes T, Smith J, et al: Cervical vasopressin compared with no premedication and blood loss during vaginal hysterectomy: a randomized controlled trial, *Obstet Gynecol* 113:313–318, 2009.

Ballard LA, Walters MD: Transvaginal mobilization and removal of ovaries and fallopian tubes after vaginal hysterectomy, *Obstet Gynecol* 87:35–39, 1996.

Cruikshank SH, Kovac SR: Randomized comparison of three surgical methods used at the time of vaginal hysterectomy to prevent posterior enterocele, *Am J Obstet Gynecol* 180:859–865, 1999.

Dicker RC, Greenspan JR, Strauss LT, et al: Complications of abdominal and vaginal hysterectomy among women of reproductive age in the United States. The collaborative review of sterilization, *Am J Obstet Gynecol* 144:841–848, 1982.

Johnson N, Barlow D, Lethaby A, et al: Surgical approach to hysterectomy for benign gynaecological disease, *Cochrane Database Syst Rev* 19(2):CD003677, 2006.

Karram MM: Vaginal hysterectomy. In Baggish MS, Karram MM, editors: *Atlas of Pelvic Anatomy and Gynecologic Surgery*, ed 2, Philadelphia, 2006, Saunders–Elsevier.

Keshavarz H, Hillis SD, Kiede BA, et al: Hysterectomy surveillance–United States, 1994-1999, *MMWR Surveill Summ* 51(SSO5):1–8, 2002.

Kovac SR: Decision-directed hysterectomy: a possible approach to improve medical and economic outcomes, *Intl J Obstet Gynaecol* 71:159–169, 2000.

Levy B, Emery L: Randomized trial of suture versus electrosurgical bipolar vessel sealing in vaginal hysterectomy, *Obstet Gynecol* 102:147–151, 2003.

Long JB, Eiland RJ, Hentz JG, et al: Randomized trial of preemptive local analgesia in vaginal surgery, *Int Urogynecol J Pelvic Floor Dysfunct* 20:5–10, 2009.

Nichols DH, Randall CL: *Vaginal surgery*, ed 2, Baltimore, 1983, Williams & Wilkins.

O'Neal MG, Beste T, Shackelford DP: Utility of preemptive local analgesia in vaginal hysterectomy, *Am J Obstet Gynecol* 189:1539–1541, 2003.

Wu JM, Wechter ME, Geller EJ, et al: Hysterectomy rates in the United States, 2003, *Obstet Gynecol* 110:1091–1095, 2007.

Surgical Procedures to Suspend a Prolapsed Uterus

5

Christopher F. Maher MD and Mickey Karram MD

 Video Clips online

5-1 Sacrospinous Hysteropexy Anterior Mesh and Posterior Repair
5-2 Sacrospinous Hysteropexy, Anterior Perigee Mesh, Posterior Repair, and Tension-Free Vaginal Tape—the Transobturator Approach
5-3 Sacrospinous Hysteropexy and Posterior Repair

5-4 Large Prolapse Suitable for Anterior and Posterior Colporrhaphy and a Sacrospinous Hysteropexy
5-5 Overactive Bladder Animation
5-6 Abdominal Sacral Colpohysteropexy (Dual-Mesh Technique)
5-7 Uphold Uterine Suspension
5-8 Uterine Prolapse with Vaginal Laceration

Uterine preservation in prolapse surgery is an attractive option for women for a variety of reasons, including the ability to retain fertility, the desire not to remove a normal organ (the perception is that the cervix is an important structure for pelvic floor stability and sexual satisfaction), and that hysteropexy is a less invasive procedure than hysterectomy with reduced blood loss and surgical time. Because the rate of hysterectomy for menorrhagia is decreasing after the introduction of progesterone-releasing intrauterine devices, all pelvic floor surgeons need to be proficient in uterine preservation techniques for the management of uterine prolapse (Figure 5-1). Table 5-1 lists the advantages and disadvantages of uterine preservation.

Women with increased risk of cervical or endometrial cancer are not candidates for uterine preservation and are excluded if they have any abnormal uterine bleeding, are taking tamoxifen for breast cancer, and have had prior cervical dysplasia abnormalities; they must be prepared to have ongoing routine gynecologic surveillance. Because 0.8% of postmenopausal women undergoing vaginal hysterectomy for prolapse have an incidental finding of endometrial cancer, it has been recommended that all women considering uterine preservation should undergo either transvaginal ultrasound assessment or a histologic assessment of the endometrium before surgery to minimize the risk of preserving a uterus with endometrial cancer (Frick et al, 2010; Renganathan, Edwards, Duckett, 2010). Box 5-1 lists the contraindications to uterine preservation surgery.

In women desiring uterine preservation, a variety of surgical options are available including the Manchester repair, vaginal sacrospinous hysteropexy, and abdominal uterosacral or sacral hysteropexy (e.g., laparoscopically, robotic, open). More recently, vaginal mesh kits such as the Uphold system (Boston Scientific) have been promoted as uterine-preserving procedures. The Manchester repair has largely been abandoned as a result of the recurrence of prolapse in excess of 20% of patients in the first few months, a decrease in fertility, pregnancy wastage as high as 50%, and future sampling of the cervix. In addition, the endometrium can be difficult to access due to vaginal re-epithelialization or cervical stenosis.

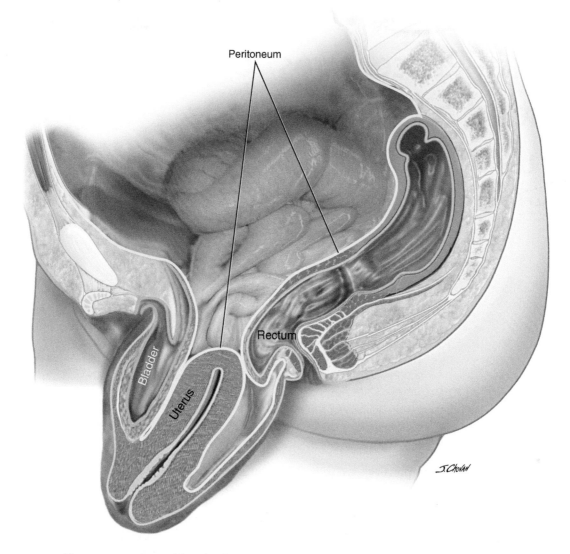

Peritoneum

Rectum

Bladder

Uterus

J. Chovan

Figure 5-1 Lateral view of the pelvis demonstrates uterine procidentia with significant bladder prolapse.

Table 5-1 Perceived and Factual Advantages and Disadvantages of Uterine-Preserving Prolapse Surgery

Advantages	Disadvantages
Retains fertility.	Retains fertility.
Retains a healthy organ.	Menses are ongoing.
Perceived role of the uterus and cervix is important in pelvic stability and sexual satisfaction.	Ongoing Gynaecological surveillance of cervix and endometrium is required.
Is a less invasive procedure.	Small, ongoing risk for cervical or endometrial cancer exists.
Reduces surgical time and blood loss.	If oopherectomy performed at hysterectomy there is no risk of ovarian cancer
Offers a quicker recovery.	Sampling cervix or endometrium is difficult.
If mesh utilised concomitantly the risk of mesh exposure is reduced at hysteropexy as compared to hysterectomy	Subsequent hysterectomy is difficult, especially if mesh is incorporated in the original prolapse surgery.
Retention of the cervix allows continuity between level 2 (native tissue or graft) and level 1 apical compartment repair.	
Outcomes are similar with hysterectomy (four case control studies).	Higher failure rate of hysteropexy in one randomized control trial, as compared with hysterectomy.

Box 5-1 Possible Contraindications for Uterine Preservation

Uterine abnormalities

Fibroids, adenomyosis, endometrial pathologic sampling

Current or recent cervical dysplasia

Abnormal menstrual bleeding

Postmenopausal bleeding

Familial cancer BRAC1 and 2 x increased risk of ovarian cancer and possibly serous endometrial cancers

Hereditary nonpolyposis colonic cancer; 40% to 50% lifetime risk for endometrial cancer

Tamoxifen therapy

Inability to comply with routine gynecologic surveillance

In four case control studies, the sacrospinous hysteropexy (Figure 5-2) was shown to be as effective as hysterectomy for the management of prolapse with a reduction in surgical time, admission time, and a quick return to activities of daily living (Maher, 2001a; Hefni et al, 2003; van Brummen et al, 2003; Dietz et al, 2007). More recently in a randomized controlled trial (RCT), Dietz and colleagues (2007) demonstrated at 12 months a significantly higher recurrence rate after hysteropexy (9 of 34; 27%), as compared with a hysterectomy group (2 of 31; 7%) ($p < 0.01$). The postoperative total vaginal length was significantly longer in the hysteropexy group, as compared with the hysterectomy group (8.8 and 7.3 cm, respectively; $p < 0.001$). The failures in this study were all grade 4 uterine prolapse. Clinicians need to be mindful of this latest result and, if verified in further studies, consider it evidence that perhaps uterine preservation in women with large procidentia should be avoided.

One traditional problem associated with sacrospinous colpopexy has been the high rate of postoperative anterior compartment prolapse. With increasing data available that support the efficacy of anterior compartment mesh augmentation, utilising anterior transvaginal mesh in women......is tempting. Hysteropexy and anterior compartment mesh is possibly further appealing when the alternative of vaginal hysterexomy and mesh procedure in a single study increased the risk of vaginal mesh erosion by a factor of 5, compared with those not undergoing hysterectomy (Collinet et al, 2006). The authors of this text recently reported their experience using anterior mesh and hysteropexy in 100 women. At 12 months, the subjective success rate of 84% was achieved with an objective success rate in all vaginal compartments of 75% with a 10% mesh erosion rate. Three women have subsequently undergone vaginal hysterectomy and vault suspension for recurrent uterine prolapse. This surgery requires further evaluation.

Only limited data are available on pregnancy outcome after sacrospinous hysteropexy in the literature. Fourteen women successfully gave birth from 15 pregnancies (1 twin); 6 women delivered by elective cesarean birth, and 9 gave birth vaginally. One in each group underwent subsequent prolapse surgery (Kovac, Cruikshank, 1993; Maher et al, 2001b).

Alternative abdominal approaches include laparoscopic suture hysteropexy and sacral hysteropexy. The plicated uterosacral ligament and cardinal ligaments are resutured to the cervix during laparoscopic suture hysteropexy (Maher, 2001a). Although the procedure is simple and safe, the objective success rate was only 79% at 12 months with the main problem being cervical elongation. The authors of this text rarely perform this technique.

The sacral hysteropexy is often suggested as the abdominal approach to uterine preservation (Table 5-2) and has been described since 1997. Because of excellent

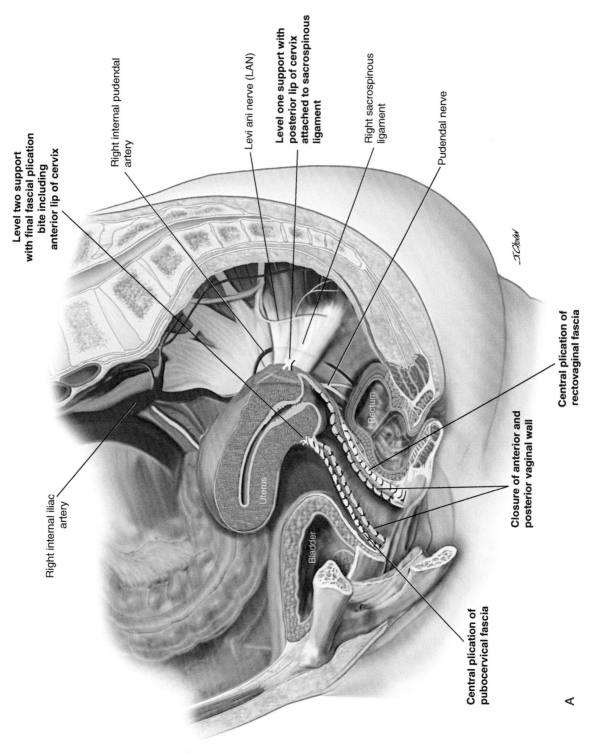

**Level two support
with final fascial plication
bite including
anterior lip of cervix**

Right internal pudendal
artery

Levi ani nerve (LAN)

**Level one support with
posterior lip of cervix
attached to sacrospinous
ligament**

Right sacrospinous
ligament

Pudendal nerve

Right internal iliac
artery

Uterus

Rectum

Bladder

**Central plication of
pubocervical fascia**

**Closure of anterior and
posterior vaginal wall**

**Central plication of
rectovaginal fascia**

A

Figure 5-2 A, Native tissue sacrospinous hysteropexy with the distal posterior cervix attached to right sacrospinous ligament (SSL) and anterior and posterior colporrhaphy are demonstrated.

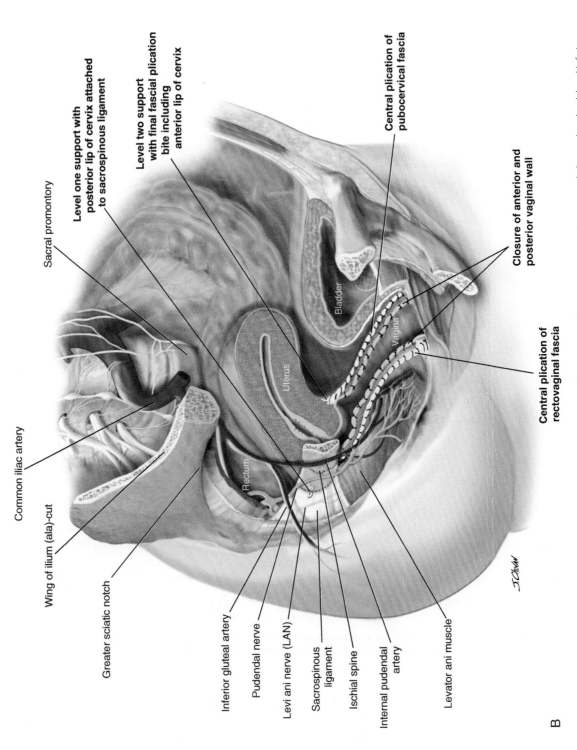

Common iliac artery

Wing of ilium (ala)-cut

Greater sciatic notch

Sacral promontory

Level one support with posterior lip of cervix attached to sacrospinous ligament

Level two support with final fascial plication bite including anterior lip of cervix

Central plication of pubocervical fascia

Bladder

Vagina

Uterus

Closure of anterior and posterior vaginal wall

Central plication of rectovaginal fascia

Rectum

Inferior gluteal artery

Pudendal nerve

Levi ani nerve (LAN)

Sacrospinous ligament

Ischial spine

Internal pudendal artery

Levator ani muscle

B

Figure 5-2, cont'd. B, Lateral view of the pelvis demonstrates the relationship of sacrospinous hysteropexy suspension to vessels (internal pudendal and inferior gluteal arteries) and pudendal and levator ani nerves.

Table 5-2 Efficacy of Abdominal Sacral Hysteropexy

Author, Year	Approach	Number	Review Months	Type of Mesh	Success Rate	
Banu, 1997	Open	19	36	Mersilene mesh fixed to the posterior uterus	100%	No complications
Leron, Stanton, 2001	Open	13	16	Teflon mesh attached to the uterine isthmus	100%	No complications
Barranger, Fritel, Pigne, 2003	Open	30	44.5	Mersuture polyester fiber attached to the anterior and posterior vagina	93%	One reoperation for uterine prolapse; three pregnancies
Costantini, 2005	Open	34	51	Mersilene mesh (polypropylene) fixed to the anterior and posterior vagina	91%	One surgery for uterine prolapse
Roovers et al, 2004	Open	32	94	Gore-Tex (polypropylene) fixed to the anterior and posterior vagina	68%	26% reoperation
Rosenblatt, 2008	Laparoscopic	40	12	Polypropylene fixed to uterosacral ligaments and posterior vagina	Mean C −4.84	
Price, 2010	Laparoscopic	51	2.5	Atrium polypropylene fixed to anterior cervix	98% Mean C −8.9	Reoperation for one uterine prolapse, five for anterior one enterocele

Table 5-3 Comparative Studies on Efficacy of Suburethral Tapes for Intrinsic Sphincter Deficiency

Study	Study Type	Numbers	ISD	Review Months	Outcomes
Miller, 2006	Retrospective	Monarc TOT: 85 TVT: 60	Borderline low MUCP (<42 cm water)	3	TOT: 6 times more likely to fail than TVT
Jeon, 2008	Retrospective	TOT: 72 TVT: 94	MUCP	24	TOT: 5 times more likely to fail than TVT
Guerette, 2008	Retrospective	TOT: 70	Compared normal and low MUCP, VLPP	8	TOT: 7 times more likely to fail if low MUCP versus normal MUCP
Gungorduk, 2009	Retrospective	TVT: 180 TOT: 120	ISD	31	TOT: 4.9 times more likely to fail than TVT
Schierlitz, 2008	Prospective RCT	TVT: 67 TOT: 71	MUCP: <20 VLPP: <60	6	TOT 2.1 times more likely to fail than TVT

ISD, Intrinsic sphincter deficiency; MUCP, maximum urethral closure pressure; RCT, randomized controlled trial; TOT, transobturator; TVT, tension-free vaginal tape; VLPP, Valsalva leak-point pressure.

outcomes with sacral colpopexy anecdotally, this procedure is gaining in popularity. Less than 180 cases with a relatively long period of review (12 to 94 months) are reported in the literature (Table 5-3). Three pregnancies have been reported, but no data on deliveries or on the impact of pregnancy or childbirth on prolapse surgery are available. Reoperation for prolapse has been reported in 10 patients. Standardization in the choice of graft and the surgical technique of attaching the graft to the uterus or vagina is distinctly lacking. Three surgeons used a single sheet of mesh attached to the posterior cervix or vagina and three used two sheets of mesh attached to the anterior and posterior vagina connected via the broad ligament. Two case series reported satisfactory outcomes after the laparoscopic approach with early follow-up and with different surgical techniques. Rosenblatt et al, 2008 attached the mesh to the uterosacral ligaments and posterior cervix, whereas Price et al, 2010 attached the mesh to the anterior cervix. The paucity of data on this technique may reflect a reluctance of surgeons to perform this relatively technical and challenging surgery when an effective vaginal approach is available; secondarily, any future hysterectomy and or prolapse surgery would be difficult.

Several authors have reported objective success rates of over 90% with sacral hysteropexy (Leron, Stanton, 2001; Barranger, Fritel, Pigne, 2003), in which mesh secures the cervix to the sacrum. In one RCT, Roover and associates (2004) compared sacral hysteropexy with vaginal hysterectomy and repair. They reported a significantly higher resurgical rate for prolapse in the hysteropexy group. Cosson has advocated uterine preservation as part of the total vaginal mesh repair because hysterectomy was an independent risk factor for mesh complications (Collinet et al, 2006); however, little data are available for total vaginal mesh with uterine preservation.

Uterine preservation at prolapse surgery is feasible, safe, and effective. The reconstructive pelvic surgeon has a variety of surgical options available that can be individualized to meet the needs of the patient.

Case 1: Sacrospinous Hysteropexy Anterior Mesh and Posterior Repair

 View: Video 5-1

A 67-year-old woman with uterine procidentia exhibited symptoms of voiding difficulties but no bowel dysfunction. No urinary tract infections were reported, and urodynamic testing before surgery demonstrated a stable bladder without stress urinary incontinence (SUI). The postvoid residual urine was 150 ml, and maximum urinary flow rate was 12 ml/sec. With the prolapse reduced, no occult stress incontinence was demonstrated.

After the various surgical options were discussed, including hysterectomy, the patient elected to undergo sacrospinous hysteropexy, anterior Prolift mesh, and posterior vaginal repair (Figure 5-3).

Surgical Steps

1. Hydrodissection with 50 ml Marcaine solution 0.25% and adrenalin floods the anterior and posterior vaginal walls.

2. A midline incision is made in the anterior vaginal mucosa, and the bladder is reflected medially from the vaginal mucosa out to the inferior pubic rami to create a paravesical space. The bladder is also mobilized from the anterior cervix.

3. The anterior Prolift mesh is introduced with care to ensure that the bladder is protected from inadvertent damage during the introduction of trocars to the paravesical spaces (see Chapter 8, Surgical Management of Anterior Vaginal Wall Prolapse). The distal tail of the mesh is secured to the anterior cervix, and the proximal mesh is fixed to the paraurethral mucosa with 2.0 Vicryl suture. Initial tensioning of the mesh is performed to ensure that the mesh sits loosely below the bladder. The anterior vaginal mucosa is closed with a continuous 2.0 Vicryl suture.

4. The posterior vaginal compartment is opened, bilaterally creating the pararectal space. The right pararectal space is bordered by the right puborectalis muscle laterally and inferiorly, the rectum medially, and the coccygeus muscle and the sacrospinous ligament (SSL) running from the ischial spine to the medial edge of the sacrum at the apex.

5. Sutures traverse the SSL 2 cm medial to the ischial spine using the Miya Hook. Usually, two sutures are loaded for each pass, and delayed absorbable 2.0 polydioxanone sutures (PDSs) are used to secure the vagina to the ligament, and a Gore-Tex permanent suture secures the distal posterior margin of the cervix to the SSL. Any permanent suture may be used for the hysteropexy suture; however, because the vaginal suture traverses the vaginal mucosa, a permanent suture may result in granulation tissue or sinus formation (or both).

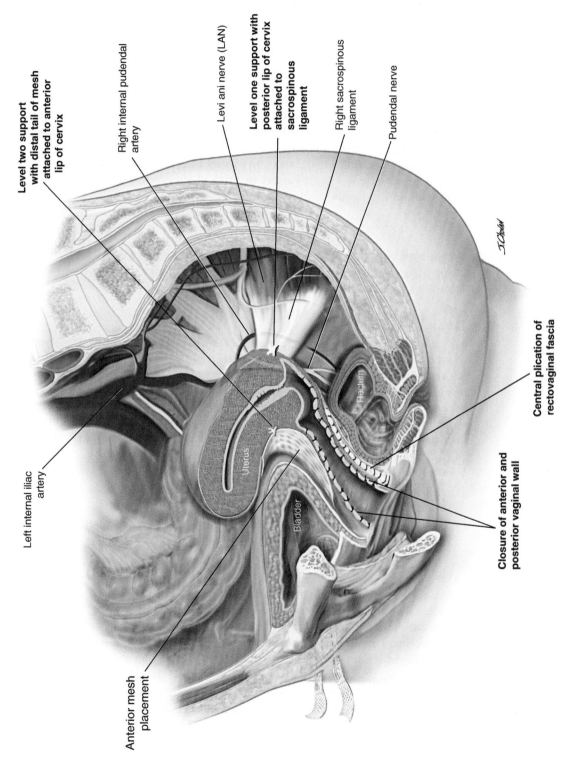

Level two support with distal tail of mesh attached to anterior lip of cervix

Right internal pudendal artery

Levi ani nerve (LAN)

Level one support with posterior lip of cervix attached to sacrospinous ligament

Right sacrospinous ligament

Pudendal nerve

Left internal iliac artery

Anterior mesh placement

Uterus

Bladder

Rectum

Closure of anterior and posterior vaginal wall

Central plication of rectovaginal fascia

Figure 5-3 Lateral aspect of the pelvis demonstrates sacrospinous hysteropexy, anterior mesh repair, and posterior colporrhaphy.

6. The rectovaginal fascia is centrally plicated with 2.0 PDSs.

7. A Gore-Tex sacrospinous suture is distally inserted through the cervix with a No. 3 Mayo needle, and a second PDS is inserted through the left and right sides of the incised vaginal mucosa.

8. The posterior vaginal mucosa is closed with 2.0 Vicryl to approximately the lower one third, and the sacrospinous hysteropexy suture is tied. The posterior vaginal mucosa is closed to the introitus, and the vaginal sacrospinous suture is tied.

9. Finally, the mesh is tensioned so it sits just below the bladder with no excessive tension on the mesh or arms. The sheath over the mesh arms are removed and the mesh is trimmed from the exit points in the groin.

10. The perineum is reconstituted.

11. A cystoscopy is performed to ensure that the bladder mucosa is intact and that the ureters are patent. A rectal examination is completed to ensure that the rectal mucosa is intact.

12. Antibiotics are initiated, thromboembolic stockings are worn for 7 days, and self-administered enoxaparin sodium (Clexane) (20 mg) is injected daily for 5 days for every patient. Patients at high risk of thromboembolic events must complete an extended course of self-administered Clexane (40 mg).

13. The vaginal pack is removed at 6:00 AM after surgery, and the indwelling catheter is removed at 12:00 PM; a trial of void is started.

See Video 5-1 for a demonstration of sacrospinous hysteropexy, anterior mesh, and posterior repair.

Case Discussion

The patient has no contraindications to uterine preservation and is happy to avoid undergoing hysterectomy to realize the benefits of reduced surgical time and blood loss. Despite the literature in four case control studies, attesting to equivalence of hysteropexy and hysterectomy, data from a single RCT reported less uterine prolapse in the hysterectomy group. Anecdotally in the authors' practice and because of recurrences in women with large and uterine dominant prolapse, encouraging hysterectomy in women with significant uterine descent (3 cm or more beyond the introitus) is now the tendency, despite the lack of any direct supporting data. Certainly, the hysteropexy remains an excellent option in women with leading anterior or posterior compartment prolapse and with the uterus not descending to the introitus.

Although the symptoms of voiding dysfunction preoperatively are unreliable, the authors routinely perform urodynamic evaluation before surgery in all women with large prolapse and in women with any symptoms of voiding difficulties to document flow rate, detrusor-voiding pressure, and residual urine. Before prolapse surgery, most women mistakenly believe that prolapse surgery will correct associated bladder symptoms. The surgeon is responsible for discussing these issues preoperatively and for informing the patient that she has a small risk of preoperative voiding symptoms persisting after surgery. Women with normal voiding preoperatively are informed of a small risk for the development of new voiding difficulties that may require clean, intermittent, postoperative self-catheterization, as stated on the procedure-specific consent form. As previously documented by the authors of this text, of the 14 women who underwent sacral colpopexy or vaginal sacrospinous colpopexy with significant stage 2 prolapse and preoperative voiding difficulties, 11 (78%) had postoperative resolution of voiding symptoms (Maher et al, 2004).

Case 2: Sacrospinous Hysteropexy, Anterior Perigee Mesh, Posterior Repair, and Tension-Free Vaginal Tape—the Transobturator Approach

View: Video 5-2

A 55-year-old woman has symptomatic uterovaginal prolapse and urinary stress incontinence. An examination with straining reveals the anterior compartment extending 2 cm beyond the introitus, cervix, and posterior compartment at the introitus with a deficient perineum. Urodynamic testing demonstrates the bladder to be stable with normal voiding and significant urinary stress incontinence with normal urethral closure pressure.

After a detailed discussion of all options, the patient is scheduled for a sacrospinous hysteropexy, Perigee anterior mesh (American Medical Systems [AMS]), and a posterior repair with remodeling perineum and transobturator sling.

Surgical Steps

1. Hydrodissection with 50 ml Marcaine solution 0.25% and adrenalin floods the anterior and posterior compartments.

2. A midline anterior vaginal incision is made from the cervix to 3 cm from the urethral meatus to ensure adequate access for the tension-free vaginal tape (TVT) using the transobturator approach at the completion of the surgery. Using sharp dissection the bladder is mobilised from the vaginal mucosa laterally to the pelvic side wall creating the paravesical space.

3. The anterior Perigee mesh is introduced into the paravesical space with caution to ensure that the bladder mucosa is not breached. The distal tail of the mesh is secured to the anterior cervix, and the proximal mesh is fixed to the paraurethral mucosa with 2.0 Vicryl suture. Initial tensioning of the mesh is performed to ensure that the mesh sits loosely below the bladder. The anterior vaginal mucosa is closed with a continuous 2.0 Vicryl suture.

4. The posterior vaginal compartment is opened, bilaterally creating the pararectal space. The right pararectal space is bordered by the right puborectalis muscle laterally and inferiorly, the rectum medially, and the coccygeus muscle and SSL running from the ischial spine to the medial edge of the sacrum at the apex.

5. Sutures are placed through the SSL 2 cm medially to the ischial spine using the Miya Hook. Usually, two sutures are loaded for each pass, and delayed absorbable 2.0 PDSs are used to secure the vagina to the ligament, and a Gore-Tex permanent suture secures the distal posterior margin of the cervix to the SSL. Any permanent suture may be used for the hysteropexy suture; however, because the vaginal suture traverses the vaginal mucosa, a permanent suture may result in granulation tissue or sinus formation (or both).

6. The rectovaginal fascia is centrally plicated using 2.0 PDSs.

7. A Gore-Tex sacrospinous suture is distally inserted through the cervix with a No. 3 Mayo needle, and a second PDS is inserted through the left and right sides of the incised vaginal mucosa.

8. The posterior vaginal mucosa is closed with 2.0 Vicryl to approximately the lower one third, and the sacrospinous hysteropexy suture is tied. The posterior vaginal mucosa is closed to the introitus, and the vaginal sacrospinous suture is tied.

9. Finally, the mesh is tensioned so it sits just below the bladder with no excessive tension on the mesh or arms. The sheath over the mesh arms are removed and the mesh is trimmed from the exit points in the groin.

10. The perineum is reconstituted.

11. TVT is inserted using the transobturator approach.

12. A cystoscopy is performed to ensure that the bladder mucosa is intact and the ureters are patent. A rectal examination is completed to ensure that the rectal mucosa is intact.

13. Antibiotics are initiated, thromboembolic stockings are worn for 7 days, and self-administered enoxaparin sodium (Clexane) (20 mg) is injected daily for 5 days for every patient. Patients at high risk of thromboembolic events must complete an extended course of self-administered Clexane (40 mg).

14. The vaginal pack is removed at 6:00 AM after surgery, and the indwelling catheter is removed at 12:00 PM; a trial of void is started.

See Video 5-2 for a demonstration of sacrospinous hysteropexy, anterior Perigee mesh, posterior repair, and tension-free vaginal tape, and the transobturator approach.

Case Discussion

This case raises several important factors. Although clinicians discuss success rates for surgery for isolated compartments, including the anterior, apical, or posterior, more than 80% of women undergoing surgery have multiple compartment prolapse, and approximately 25% also have concomitant urinary stress incontinence that they want addressed. Many researchers report the success rate in the isolated compartment that is under evaluation, and some report a success rate for each compartment; however, the more meaningful data for patients are the success rates for which this surgery can be incorporated into the overall pelvic floor repair and the objective success rates at all vaginal sites in total.

The treatment of SUI with normal urethral resistance is a second issue worthy of discussion. The authors of this text routinely use transobturator suburethral tapes; the success rate appears equal to that of the classical retropubic tape with less morbidity. Growing evidence suggests that in women who are undergoing vaginal surgery with intrinsic sphincter deficiency (ISD), SUI, and prolapse, the classic retropubic tape should be used (see Table 5-3). Importantly, all studies have used Monarc transobturator sling as the transobturator tape; to date, comparative studies of TVT–transobturator approach in women with ISD are not available.

Case 3: Sacrospinous Hysteropexy and Posterior Repair

 View: Video 5-3

A 48-year-old woman has posterior compartment prolapse extending 2 cm beyond the introitus, causing impaired defecation. Vaginal digitation is regularly used to complete defecation. She has associated urinary frequency and urgency, and urodynamic testing has confirmed bladder overactivity and normal voiding. Her cervical screening is normal, and her menses are regular. An examination reveals the anterior compartment was well supported with the cervix extending to the mid-vagina, and the bimanual examination confirms that the uterus is mobile, anteverted, and of normal size. The patient wants to preserve her uterus and has no contraindications to hysteropexy. Thus she gives consent for sacrospinous hysteropexy and posterior repair (Figure 5-4).

Surgical Steps

1. Hydrodissection with 50 ml Marcaine solution 0.25% with adrenalin floods the posterior vaginal compartment.

2. A midline incision opens the posterior vaginal mucosa from introitus to cervix.

3. Sharp dissection of the rectum from the vaginal mucosa bilaterally opens the pararectal space. The right pararectal space is bordered by the right puborectalis muscle laterally and inferiorly, the rectum medially, and the coccygeus muscle and SSL running from the ischial spine to the medial edge of the sacrum at the apex.

4. Sutures traverse the SSL using the Miya Hook. Usually, two sutures are loaded for each pass, and delayed absorbable 2.0 PDSs are used to secure the vagina to the ligament, and a Gore-Tex permanent suture secures the distal posterior margin of the cervix to the SSL. Any permanent suture may be used for the hysteropexy suture; however, because the vaginal suture traverses the vaginal mucosa, a permanent suture may result in granulation tissue or sinus formation (or both).

5. The rectovaginal fascia is centrally plicated with 2.0 PDSs.

6. A Gore-Tex sacrospinous suture is fixed to the distal posterior cervix with a No. 3 Mayo needle, and a second PDS is inserted through the left and right sides of the upper vaginal mucosa.

7. The posterior vagina mucosa is closed with 2.0 Vicryl to approximately the lower one third, and the sacrospinous hysteropexy suture is tied. The posterior vaginal mucosa is closed to the introitus, and the vaginal sacrospinous suture is tied.

8. The perineum is reconstituted.

9. A rectal examination is completed to ensure that the rectal mucosa is intact.

10. Antibiotics are initiated, thromboembolic stockings are worn for 7 days, and self-administered enoxaparin sodium (Clexane) (20 mg) is injected daily for 5 days for every patient. Patients at high risk of thromboembolic events must complete an extended course of self-administered Clexane (40 mg).

11. The vaginal pack is removed at 6:00 AM after surgery, and the indwelling catheter is removed at 12:00 PM; a trial of void is started

See Video 5-3 for a demonstration of sacrospinous hysteropexy with posterior repair and perineal reconstruction.

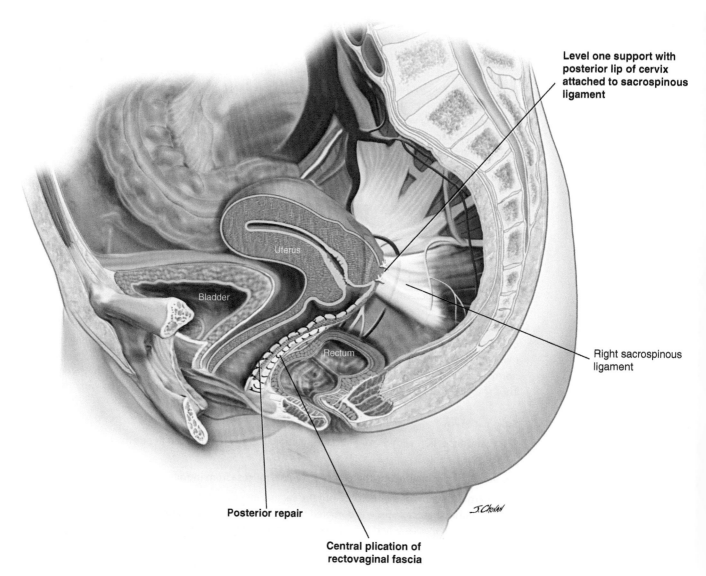

Level one support with posterior lip of cervix attached to sacrospinous ligament

Right sacrospinous ligament

Uterus

Bladder

Rectum

Posterior repair

Central plication of rectovaginal fascia

J. Chovan

Figure 5-4 Sacrospinous hysteropexy and posterior colporrhaphy are visualized in this lateral view. The distal posterior cervix is attached to the sacrospinous ligament (SSL), and suture plication of the posterior vaginal wall is performed.

Case Discussion

This case highlights the importance of the surgeon having a variety of surgical options available and individualizing them, depending on the patient's history, examination, and preferences. Certainly, hysterectomy or vaginal mesh is not required in many patients as illustrated in **Video 5-4, "Large Prolapse Suitable for Anterior and Posterior Colporrhaphy and a Sacrospinous Hysteropexy."**

This case also promotes a discussion on the common association of bladder overactivity and pelvic organ prolapse (POP). Without exception, patients undergoing prolapse surgery presume that the prolapse surgery will have a beneficial effect on bladder symptoms and are disappointed if these bladder overactivity symptoms persist or worsen after surgery.

Traditional teaching states that the overactive bladder (OAB) is a functional problem of poor storage and compliance as demonstrated in **Video 5-5, "Overactive Bladder Animation,"** and is unrelated to anatomic issues such as prolapse. In the authors' unit, 28% of women undergoing prolapse surgery have bladder overactivity, and approximately one third have resolution of these symptoms after prolapse surgery, which is consistent in both vaginal and abdominal procedures (Maher et al, 2004). Finally, 10% of women develop *de novo* bladder overactivity after prolapse surgery. A recent comprehensive review by de Boer and associates (2010) on the association of OAB and POP noted the following:

- OAB is twice as common in women with prolapse as in women without prolapse.

- Bladder overactivity occurs in 50% of women undergoing prolapse surgery.

- Impact of POP surgery varies widely; women are 1.8 times more likely to have OAB symptoms before POP surgery than after.

- Vaginal pessaries that correct prolapse also result in a reduction of OAB symptoms.

- Bladder obstruction may have role in the pathophysiologic characteristics of OAB.

- No correlation exists between prolapse compartment and OAB.

- It is unclear which patients will have resolution, persistence, or *de novo* development of OAB symptoms.

The preoperative emphasis of counseling of patients with OAB is that POP is an anatomic defect and OAB is a functional derangement issue. Anatomic correction of prolapse does not usually result in a resolution of OAB symptoms, and that anticholinergic medications and bladder retraining will be required after prolapse surgery. In patients who do not have an OAB before surgery, 5% to 10% will develop these symptoms after prolapse surgery. A vital role of preoperative counseling is to ensure that the patient has realistic expectations of the surgical outcomes.

Case 4: Abdominal Sacral Colpohysteropexy

 View: Video 5-6

A 32-year-old Caucasian woman has symptomatic advanced POP. An examination confirms that the majority of the prolapse is stemming from the anterior segment, which descends 4 cm beyond the introitus when she strains in a supine position. In addition, the cervix descends just beyond the hymen with straining. The posterior vaginal wall is relatively well supported. Further examination identifies a cervix of fairly normal length, and the bimanual examination reveals a normal size uterus. The patient has no contraindications to uterine preservation.

She denies any urinary incontinence or voiding dysfunction. Filling cystometric testing notes a stable detrusor to a maximum capacity of 450 ml with no evidence of occult SUI. She is symptomatic with her prolapse and desires definitive therapy. Although she is not interested in future fertility, the patient is insistent on preserving her uterus. She is consulted and consents to a laparoscopic sacral colpohysteropexy (Figure 5-5) using a dual-mesh technique (Figure 5-6).

Surgical Steps

1. Abdominal insufflation and the placement of trocars are performed.

2. To perform the dual-mesh technique, two pieces of mesh are used; one is placed in a conventional fashion along the posterior vaginal wall and back of the cervix and brought to the sacral promontory; the second piece of mesh is cut in such a way that it measures approximately 4.5 cm wide with two arms extending approximately 11 cm (see Figure 5-6). The specific dimensions of the mesh need to be tailored to the size of the particular cervix of the patient.

3. After mobilization of the bladder off the anterior portion of the cervix, two windows are created in the broad ligament. These are generated under direct visualization, ensuring no disruption of the uterine vessels, as well as maintaining an awareness of the exact location of the ureter on each side. Once these windows are made, the peritoneal reflection is extended toward the round ligament on each side. The main part of the anterior mesh is then fixed with numerous sutures to the anterior vaginal wall and anterior portions of the cervix, making sure that the bladder has been appropriately mobilized in a caudal direction, which should always be sharply done if the patient has had previous cesarean sections.

4. The arms of the mesh are then tunneled through the window of the broad ligament and brought back and fixed to the sacral promontory in the same area (usually at the level of S3) that the posterior mesh is fixed.

5. The remainder of the procedure is as would be performed for an open abdominal sacral colpohysteropexy. **(See Video 5-6, "Abdominal Sacral Colpohysteropexy [Dual-Mesh Technique]" for a demonstration of abdominal sacral colpohysteropexy.** 📹**)**

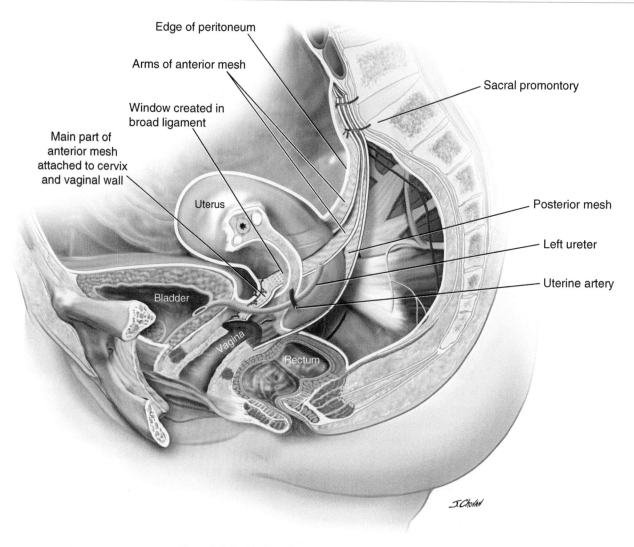

Edge of peritoneum

Arms of anterior mesh

Window created in broad ligament

Main part of anterior mesh attached to cervix and vaginal wall

Uterus

Bladder

Vagina

Rectum

Sacral promontory

Posterior mesh

Left ureter

Uterine artery

J. CHOVAN

Figure 5-5 Dual-leaf sacral colpohysteropexy is represented.

Case Discussion

The procedure described is a relatively new procedure with no real scientific validity to date. It has been the empiric experience of the authors of this text, however, that the dual-mesh technique provides significant anterior vaginal wall support and support to the anterior cervix that was not being achieved when a single piece of mesh was posteriorly used for sacral colpohysteropexy.

The impact of this procedure on future fertility and other potential complications related to the arms and anterior placement is yet to be determined. Finally, clinicians are also performing subtotal hysterectomy and sacral colpopexy (Figure 5-7). This approach potentially avoids the risk of mesh exposure associated with performing abdominal hysterectomy and sacral colpopexy in those with uterine prolapse. The safety and efficacy of this approach requires further evaluation. Any surgery subsequently requiring the removal of the cervix could be problematic.

Case 5: Uphold Uterine Suspension

 View: Video 5-7

A 43-year-old woman (gravida 3, para 2) reports a 3-year history of progressive vaginal bulging and pressure, exacerbated by prolonged standing and exercise. Her examination reveals a fourth-degree cystocele (Point Ba +3), uterine prolapse to the introitus (C = 0), second-degree rectocele (Point Bp

Peritoneal closure over mesh

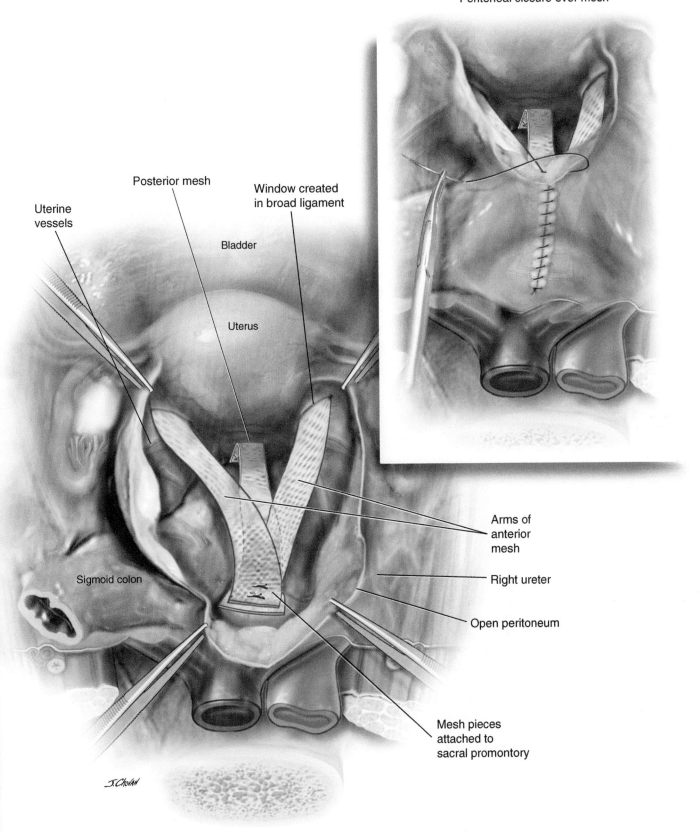

Posterior mesh

Window created
in broad ligament

Uterine
vessels

Bladder

Uterus

Sigmoid colon

Arms of
anterior
mesh

Right ureter

Open peritoneum

Mesh pieces
attached to
sacral promontory

J. Chovan

Figure 5-6 The two arms of the anterior leaf of mesh are highlighted exiting the broad ligament. They are secured with the posterior leaf to the sacral promontory. The retroperitoneal space is shown being closed over the mesh arms *(inset)*.

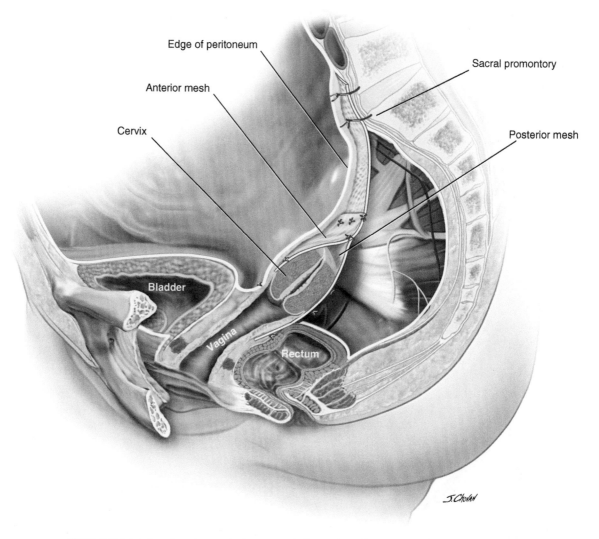

Figure 5-7 A sacral cervicocolpopexy is demonstrated after a subtotal hysterectomy for uterine prolapse.

−1) with no associated defecatory symptoms. Bimanual examination reveals a small anteverted uterus; the cervix is small but not elongated. The patient reports rare episodes of SUI, and urodynamic testing confirms the condition with a maximum urethral closure pressure (MUCP) of 48 cm H_2O. Her history is unremarkable, including no history of ovarian, uterine, or breast cancer. The patient declines pessary management and further observation and expresses interest in exploring "uterine-sparing" surgical options, if possible.

Detailed counseling with this patient includes a discussion of the risks and benefits of uterine preservation versus a traditional vaginal hysterectomy and repair and the risks and potential benefits of a mesh-augmented repair, particularly with respect to her advanced cystocele and apical defect. She expresses a clear understanding of the issues and elects to proceed with sacrospinous hysteropexy, including anterior-apical mesh augmentation using the Uphold vaginal support system (Figure 5-8).

Surgical Steps

1. Hydrodissection with at least 30 ml vasoconstrictive solution is performed. The authors of this text tend to administer 10 ml bupivacaine 0.25% with epinephrine injected in the direction of each SSL and 10 ml used in the central portion of the cystocele, from the bladder neck to vaginal apex–cervical junction.

2. A horizontal incision is made at the level of the bladder neck, rather than at the level of the standard vertical vaginal incision. This level prevents an overlap of the mesh implant and the vaginal incision and may be one factor underlying the low mesh exposure rates observed so far after this procedure.

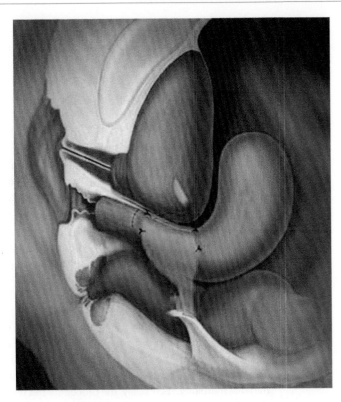

Figure 5-8 The Uphold vaginal support system.

(Image Courtesy of Boston Scientific Corporation. Opinions expressed are those of the author alone and not of Boston Scientific.)

3. Using Metzenbaum scissors, the anterior vaginal wall is dissected from the bladder. As with any mesh procedure, creating a thin vaginal flap must be avoided; in other words, an adequate amount of connective tissue should be left on the vagina to reduce the risk of postoperative mesh exposure. Sharp scissor dissection is typically carried out until the dissection has extended laterally to the descending pubic ramus on each side.

4. The SSLs are identified and palpated through the anterior approach, which may involve a combination of blunt and sharp dissections, scissor-spreading technique, or sometimes the use of the back end of a long tissue forceps as a blunt dissecting tool. The key to achieving an easy and hemostatic anterior approach to the SSL is to *maintain steady lateral pressure against the pelvic sidewall (obturator muscle)* while sweeping the paravaginal-paravesical tissues away from their lateral attachments. The surgeon's finger should be flush against the obturator muscle, maintaining constant lateral pressure and ensuring that no intervening tissue planes remain on the muscle surface. The surgeon's finger is then directed cephalad and posterior toward the bony landmark of the ischial spine.

5. Once the ischial spine is palpated, the finger is used to sweep medially, clearing a two-fingerbreadth target on the ligament. The internal finger now retracts the bladder medially. The Capio needle driver, loaded with the Uphold mesh, is inserted into the tunnel that is located between the internal finger and the pelvic sidewall.

6. The head of the Capio device is placed against the SSL-coccygeus complex, approximately 2 fingerbreadths directly medial to the ischial spine. To avoid injury to the pudendal neurovascular structures, the sutures are made into, not over, the SSL. After completing this single fixation into each SSL, no further deep pelvic surgery is needed. The Uphold procedure involves only one fixation point on each side.

7. An anterior colporrhaphy may now be performed at the surgeon's discretion. The authors' practice is to perform a simple anterior colporrhaphy (using 0-Vicryl mattress sutures) for any cases involving a significant midline cystocele, which tends to shrink the anatomic area that needs to be covered by the mesh, allowing the surgeon to use the smaller Uphold mesh for even advanced prolapse cases.

8. Tensioning the mesh arms is done to draw the mesh closer to the repair. Using 2-0 Vicryl interrupted sutures, the proximal mesh edge is tacked to the paracervical ring or to the vaginal apex, if the uterus is absent. After removing all Allis clamps and self-retaining retractor hooks, the mesh arms may now be fully tensioned until the cervix and vaginal apex are fully suspended. With a finger in the vagina, the tension of the mesh arms is checked; a definitive cephalad lift of the vaginal apex should be felt with no excessive tension in the mesh arms. The arms can be loosened, if needed, by gently pushing against them in a cephalad direction.

9. Once the tensioning of the mesh arms is confirmed and believed to be optimal, the plastic sheaths overlying the mesh are removed by clipping one of the two monofilament sutures observed running through the plastic sheath and tugging the suture-sheath assembly until it disengages. These disposable portions are discarded.

10. Using 2-0 Vicryl sutures, the distal (superior) mesh edge is tacked to ensure that it is secure just beneath the horizontal incision. The incision is now closed, and the repair is complete. A rectocele and/or sling repair, when clinically indicated, is performed after the Uphold procedure. **(See Video 5-7, "Uphold Uterine Suspension," for a demonstration of the Uphold repair.** **).**

Case Discussion

This patient's presentation is a fairly common clinical picture with a large anterior defect and a significant apical defect including uterine descent. She strongly prefers uterine preservation, if it offers good results. The authors' experience with the Uphold vaginal support system (Boston Scientific) over the past 2 years suggests that successful results can indeed be achieved with minimal morbidity. Technically, the procedure has few steps and involves relatively minimal dissection. It requires only a single apical fixation on each side and eliminates the passage of mesh through the levator muscles. When compared with the standard vaginal hysterectomy with repair, surgical times for the technique are short and recovery is quick. The overall mesh load is substantially reduced, in comparison with most other vaginal mesh repairs, and is consistent with a "minimal mesh" philosophy. Using a horizontal incision technique, the rate of mesh exposure seems to be less than reported with other mesh repairs. The Uphold repair with the uterus *in situ* should not be performed when uterine or cervical enlargement exists; hysterectomy will provide a more durable repair. Long-term follow-up and comparative trials to native tissue and other mesh repairs are required to determine whether these encouraging preliminary outcomes are maintained over time.

Case 6: Ulcerated Uterine Procidentia

View: Video 5-8

A 74-year-old woman is referred with uterine procidentia and ulceration (see Figure 5-9). Ring pessaries were previously extruded on two occasions. Clearly, having the ulceration preoperatively corrected by having the prolapse reduced is preferable. This correction would serve to decrease associated infection and urinary sepsis, as well as increase the thickness and health of the vaginal mucosa, which would be important, especially if a vaginal mesh is to be introduced. Rejuvenation of the keratinized skin observed in large procidentia to more normal mucosa is also associated with decreased bleeding on incision.

A reduction of large prolapse with ulceration and keratinized epithelium is best attempted with the patient in hospital, with an indwelling catheter draining the bladder, and the rectum emptied with a suppository. After the patient has showered and is lying in the Trendelenburg position for several hours and after the application of lidocaine gel, the prolapse is reduced and the two largest pessaries that will fit are inserted.

If the pessaries are not extruded, then the surgery is scheduled for the following month. If the pessaries are extruded with mobilization, then the clinician can elect to perform the colpocleisis procedure with the ulceration present. If the clinician is performing the repair with the introduction of mesh, a vaginal pack is inserted under general anesthesia and the vagina is closed with interrupted sutures with an indwelling catheter (IDC) in situ for 10 days. Antibiotics are commenced;

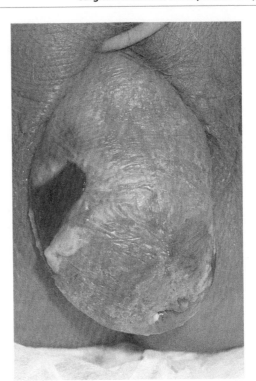

Figure 5-9 Large ulcerated uterine procidentia.

when the patient is returned to surgery for the removal of the pack and for prolapse correction, the ulceration will be healed and the vaginal epithelium will be less edematous and free of infection.

Smaller breaches of the vaginal mucosa **(see Video 5-8, "Uterine Prolapse with Vaginal Laceration."** 🎦) can occur; in this patient, the vaginal mucosa was damaged by the patient's nails as she repeatedly reduced the prolapse to void. Despite instigating the double-ring pessaries, these quickly extruded. Because the vaginal mucosa was quite healthy, the author of this text elected to proceed with the surgery with the vaginal mucosa unhealed.

SUMMARY OF SURGICAL PROCEDURES TO SUSPEND A PROLAPSED UTERUS

- As hysterectomy numbers for menorrhagia reduce the number of women presenting with uterine prolapse will increase.
- Hysteropexy is an attractive option for many women; it offers reduced surgical time, low blood loss, and a quick recovery.
- Strict suitability criteria for uterine preservation are described.
- Vaginal hysteropexy is likely as successful as hysterectomy; however, a recent single RCT demonstrated a poor anatomic outcome when hysteropexy was performed. Anecdotally, women with large uterine dominant prolapse may have a lower risk of recurrence if hysterectomy is performed. Further evaluation is required.
- Vaginal hysteropexy is well described and reported.
- Abdominal sacral hysteropexy has limited cases in the literature with a wide variation of technique.

Suggested Readings

Barranger E, Fritel X, Pigne A: Abdominal sacrohysteropexy in young women with uterovaginal prolapse: long-term follow-up, *Am J Obstet Gynecol* 189(5):1245–1250, 2003.

Banu LF: Synthetic sling for genital prolapse in young women, *Int J Gynaecol Obstet* 57(1):57–64, 1997.

Collinet P, Belot F, Debodinance P, et al: Transvaginal mesh technique for pelvic organ prolapse repair: mesh exposure management and risk factors, *Int Urogynecol J Pelvic Floor Dysfunct* 17(4):315–320, 2006.

Costantini E, Mearini L, Bini V, et al: Uterus preservation in surgical correction of urogenital prolapse, *Eur Urol* 48(4):642–649, 2005.

de Boer TA, Salvatore S, Cardozo L, et al: Pelvic organ prolapse and overactive bladder, *Neurourol Urodyn* 29(1):30–39, 2010.

Dietz V, de Jong J, Huisman M, et al: The effectiveness of the sacrospinous hysteropexy for the primary treatment of uterovaginal prolapse, *Int Urogynecol J Pelvic Floor Dysfunct* 18(11):1271–1276, 2007.

eon MJ, Jung HJ, Chung SM, et al: Comparison of the treatment outcome of pubovaginal sling, tension-free vaginal tape, and transobturator tape for stress urinary incontinence with intrinsic sphincter deficiency, *Am J Obstet Gynecol* 199(1):76e1–4, 2008.

Frick AC, Walters MD, Larkin KS, et al: Risk of unanticipated abnormal gynecologic pathology at the time of hysterectomy for uterovaginal prolapse, *Am J Obstet Gynecol* 202(5):507.e1–507.e4, 2010.

Guerette NL, Bena JF, Davila GW: Transobturator slings for stress incontinence: using urodynamic parameters to predict outcomes, *Int Urogynecol J Pelvic Floor Dysfunct* 19(1):97–102, 2008.

Gungorduk K, Celebi I, Ark C, et al: Which type of mid-urethral sling procedure should be chosen for treatment of stress urinary incontinance with intrinsic sphincter deficiency? Tension-free vaginal tape or transobturator tape, *Acta Obstet Gynecol Scand* 88(8):920–926, 2009.

Hefni M, El-Toukhy T, Bhaumik J, et al: Sacrospinous cervicocolpopexy with uterine conservation for uterovaginal prolapse in elderly women: an evolving concept, *Am J Obstet Gynecol* 188(3):645–650, 2003.

Kovac SR, Cruikshank SH: Successful pregnancies and vaginal deliveries after sacrospinous uterosacral fixation in five of nineteen patients, *Am J Obstet Gynecol* 168(6 Pt 1):1778–1783, 1993.

Leron E, Stanton SL: Sacrohysteropexy with synthetic mesh for the management of uterovaginal prolapse, *BJOG* 108(6):629–633, 2001.

Maher CF, Carey MP, Murray CJ: Laparoscopic suture hysteropexy for uterine prolapse, *Obstet Gynecol* 97(6):1010–1014, 2001a.

Maher CF, Cary MP, Slack MC, et al: Uterine preservation or hysterectomy at sacrospinous colpopexy for uterovaginal prolapse? *Int Urogynecol J Pelvic Floor Dysfunct* 12(6):381–384, 2001b.

Maher CF, Qatawneh AM, Dwyer PL, et al: Abdominal sacral colpopexy or vaginal sacrospinous colpopexy for vaginal vault prolapse: a prospective randomized study, *Am J Obstet Gynecol* 190(1):20–26, 2004.

Miller JJ, Botros SM, Akl MN, et al: Is transobturator tape as effective as tension-free vaginal tape in patients with borderline maximum urethral closure pressure? *Am J Obstet Gynecol* 195(6):1799–1804, 2006.

Price N, Slack A, Jackson SR: Laparoscopic hysteropexy: the initial results of a uterine suspension procedure for uterovaginal prolapse, *BJOG* 117(1):62–68, 2010.

Renganathan AR, Edwards R, Duckett JR: Uterus conserving prolapse surgery—what is the chance of missing a malignancy? *Int Urogynecol J* 21(7):819–821, 2010.

Roovers JP, van der Vaart CH, van der Bom JG, et al: A randomised controlled trial comparing abdominal and vaginal prolapse surgery: effects on urogenital function, *BJOG* 111(1):50–56, 2004.

Rosenblatt PL, Chelmow D, Ferzandi TR: Laparoscopic sacrocervicopexy for the treatment of uterine prolapse: a retrospective case series report, *J Minim Invasive Gynecol* 15(3):268–272, 2008.

van Brummen HJ, van de Pol G, Aalders CL, et al: Sacrospinous hysteropexy compared to vaginal hysterectomy as primary surgical treatment for a descensus uteri: effects on urinary symptoms, *Int Urogynecol J Pelvic Floor Dysfunct* 14(5):350–355, 2003.

Robot-Assisted Laparoscopic Colposacropexy and Cervicosacropexy

6

Catherine A. Matthews MD

 Video Clips online

6-1 Dissection of the Sacral Promontory
6-2 Dissection of the Rectovaginal and Vesicovaginal Space
6-3 Attachment of Anterior Mesh

6-4 Attachment of Posterior Mesh
6-5 Attachment of Mesh to the Promontory

In recent years, there has been a growing recognition that adequate support of the vaginal apex is an essential component of a durable surgical repair for pelvic organ prolapse. (Summers et al, 2006; Maher et al, 2007) Sacrocolpopexy is considered the gold standard of surgical procedures for the repair of Level I pelvic support defects with excellent long-term results. (Sullivan, Longaker, Lee, 2001; Culligan et al, 2002) Vaginal reconstructive surgical options, such as uterosacral and sacrospinous ligament suspensions and vaginally placed mesh procedures, are alternative treatments but have different effectiveness levels and are associated with different complications. Although a small number of surgeons are able to accomplish sacrocolpopexies using standard laparoscopic techniques, the majority of these procedures are performed via laparotomy because of the challenges encountered with extensive suturing and knot tying. Small case series have demonstrated similar outcomes using a laparoscopic approach with the additional benefits of reduced pain, postoperative time for recovery, and length of hospital stay. (Nezhat, Nezhat, Nezhat, 1994; Ross, 1997; Cosson et al, 2002) With the introduction of the da Vinci robot, the feasibility of more surgeons performing this operation through minimally invasive techniques has greatly expanded. The steep learning curve that is inherent in mastering intracorporeal knot tying and suturing using standard laparoscopy is greatly diminished by the use of articulating instruments, making it an accessible option for all gynecologic surgeons treating women with pelvic organ prolapse. In this chapter, the steps involved in completing a robotic-assisted colposacropexy using a Y-shaped polypropylene mesh graft are described.

Surgical Preparation and Set-Up

The patient completes a preoperative bowel preparation using two bottles of magnesium citrate and clear liquids 1 day before surgery. Although mechanical bowel cleansing has not been shown to decrease operative morbidity, the ease of sigmoid manipulation and retraction may be facilitated. Perioperative antibiotics are administered 30 minutes before the procedure, and subcutaneous heparin (5000 units) is

Case 1: Dissection of the Sacral Promontory

A 65-year-old, sexually active, Caucasian woman complains of a bothersome vaginal bulge that interferes with her ability to exercise comfortably. She denies symptoms of urinary or fecal incontinence but reports difficulty with bowel evacuation, frequently needing to splint the perineum to defecate. A total abdominal hysterectomy and Burch procedure was performed 15 years before for abnormal uterine bleeding and symptomatic stress urinary incontinence. An examination reveals a body mass index of 27, a midline vertical incision that extends to her umbilicus, a stage III vaginal vault prolapse, and a stage II distal posterior wall prolapse. Preoperative urodynamic testing reveals no evidence of recurrent stress urinary incontinence. Considering her age, level of physical activity, sexual function, and type of prolapse, the patient is counseled to undergo a robotic sacrocolpopexy with polypropylene mesh and vaginal posterior repair.

injected en route to the surgical suite for thromboprophylaxis. The patient is placed in the dorsal lithotomy position with the buttocks extending one inch over the end of the surgical table, which is covered with egg-crate to avoid slipping while in the steep Trendelenburg position. After the patient is prepped and draped, a Foley catheter is placed into the bladder and EEA sizers are inserted into the vagina and rectum. A surgical assistant is seated between the patient's legs to provide adequate vaginal and rectal manipulation during the procedure.

Surgical Technique
(Appropriate port placement and docking of the robot)

1. Pneumoperitoneum is obtained with a Veress needle technique, followed by the placement of five trocars (Figure 6-1). In a patient with prior abdominal surgery, we recommend entry in the left upper quadrant at Palmer's point. Careful port placement is integral to the success of this procedure because of the following: (1) Inadequate distances between the robotic arms and the camera results in arm collisions and interference. (2) Easy visualization and access to the sacral promontory may be compromised if the camera is inserted too low on the anterior abdominal wall. (3) If the fourth arm is not at least 3 cm above the anterior superior iliac spine (ASIS), successful bowel retraction may be compromised. When evaluating the abdomen before trocar insertion, the authors of this text have determined that at least 15 cm is required between the pubic bone and the umbilicus to rely on this landmark for the 12-mm camera port. If this distance is shorter, as it is in many women who are obese, then insertion above the umbilicus is necessary. An accessory 12-mm port, which is used for the introduction of the sutures and the mesh graft, is placed approximately 10 cm lateral and 4 cm cephalad to the camera in the right upper quadrant. An 8-mm robotic port is placed in the right lower quadrant 10 cm lateral to the accessory port and approximately 3 cm above the ASIS. The third and fourth robotic arms are placed 10 cm apart in the left lower quadrant, with the fourth arm typically as far lateral as possible.

2. After placing the patient in a steep Trendelenburg position and locking the bed, the robot is docked from the patient's left side at a 45-degree angle to the bed. Side-docking permits easy access to the vagina for the evaluation of graft tension and for the completion of the cystoscopy to ensure ureteral and bladder integrity. Care should be taken to ensure that the spine of the robot is positioned right next to the bed at the level of the patient's hip; driving it up too high, relative to the abdomen, can compromise the mobility of the fourth arm. In addition, if the robot is not close enough to the bed, then the reach of the first (right) arm may be limited. Before starting the procedure, ensuring that the bowel is not obscuring the operative field

Figure 6-1 Port placement: C, camera; A, accessory port; 1, right arm (monopolar shears); 2, left arm (PK Dissector); 3, fourth arm (Cadiere bowel retractor).

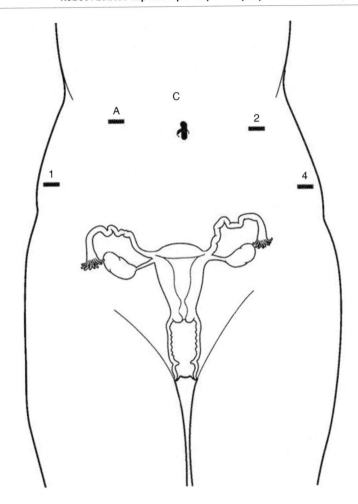

is critical, and efforts to correct this position at the beginning of the procedure can minimize frustration.

3. Necessary instruments include monopolar scissors that are introduced through the right arm, a bipolar PK dissector through the left arm, and an atraumatic bowel grasper such as a Cadiere bowel retractor that is placed through the fourth arm. The bedside assistant stands on the right side of the patient with access to a long Maryland dissector and a suction and irrigation device.

Technique of the Sacrocolpopexy Procedure

The approach is modeled exactly after the open surgical technique, which is critical to the success of a robotic-assisted laparoscopic approach to colposacropexy.

1. With the use of a 0- or 30-degree down scope, the sigmoid colon is retracted laterally using the Cadiere forceps and the right ureter is identified. When first attempting this procedure, identifying the sacral promontory with the use of a standard laparoscopic instrument with haptic feedback may be helpful before docking the robot.

2. The peritoneum overlying the sacral promontory is elevated and opened using monopolar cautery. The fat pad overlying the anterior longitudinal ligament is exposed and gently dissected away (Figure 6-2). **(See Video 6-1, "Dissection of the Sacral Promontory."**) The middle sacral artery is frequently visualized and can be coagulated using the PK dissector, if necessary.

3. A retroperitoneal tunnel is made from the sacral promontory to the level of the rectovaginal peritoneal reflection along the right paracolic gutter. **(See Video 6-1, "Dissection of the Sacral Promontory."**) The creation of this tunnel allows

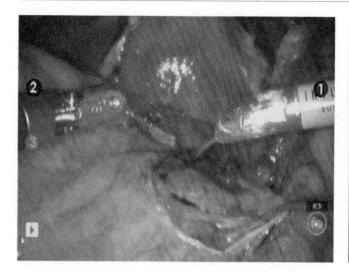

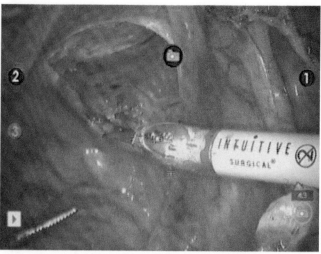

Figure 6-2 Peritoneum is opened at the sacral promontory, and the fat pad is dissected to reveal the anterior longitudinal ligament.

Figure 6-3 Peritoneal incision is extended along the cul-de-sac to the posterior vaginal wall in a T-shaped configuration to access the rectovaginal space. When performing a cervicosacropexy, developing this surgical plane is easiest before amputation of the cervix.

the sacral arm of the mesh to lie flat and decreases the time at the end of the procedure to extraperitonealize the mesh. Care must be taken to keep this tunnel just beneath the peritoneum; bleeding can be encountered in the deeper fat plane.

4. With the vagina deviated anteriorly and the rectum posteriorly using the EEA sizers, the rectovaginal space is easily identified; and the peritoneal incision is extended transversely in a T shape to expose the posterior vaginal wall (Figure 6-3). **(See Video 6-2, "Dissection of the Rectovaginal and Vesicovaginal Space."**) If indicated, the rectovaginal space can be dissected all the way down to the perineal body.

5. The vagina is then deviated posteriorly to facilitate the dissection of the bladder from the anterior vaginal wall using monopolar cautery. **(See Video 6-2, "Dissection of the Rectovaginal and Vesicovaginal Space."**) If significant scarring is encountered between the bladder and vagina, then the bladder can be retrograde filled with 300 ml saline, mixed with methylene blue dye to help identify the surgical plane. Depending on the degree of anterior vaginal wall prolapse, approximately 6 to 8 cm of anterior vaginal wall is exposed. An attempt is made to leave the peritoneum intact at the apex of the vagina to reduce the chance of mesh erosion.

6. After measuring the respective lengths of the exposed anterior and posterior vaginal walls, a correctly sized Y-shaped polypropylene graft is created by suturing together two strips of Gynemesh that are approximately 3 cm in width. Significant variability in the relative dimensions of the anterior and posterior segments of mesh can exist, thus the recommendation to fashion the graft after completing the dissection. After assessing the differences in graft placement and manipulation by suturing the two arms together before or after intracorporeal placement, the opinion of the authors of this text is that the former method is far easier. IntePro (American Medical Systems, Minnetonka, Minnesota), Alyte (Bard Medical, Covington, Georgia), and Restorelle Y (Mpathy, Raynham, Massachusetts) are preformed type 1 polypropylene Y-mesh products that are available at a higher cost.

7. The mesh graft is introduced through the accessory port after exchanging the scissors and PK dissector for a suture cut and a large needle driver. The bladder is retracted using the fourth arm, and the anterior mesh arm is placed over the anterior vaginal wall and sutured in place using 2-0 Gore-Tex sutures on CT-2 needles that are each cut to 6 inches long. Anchoring the two distal corners first (Figure 6-4), **(see Video 6-3, "Attachment of Anterior Mesh"**) and then placing a

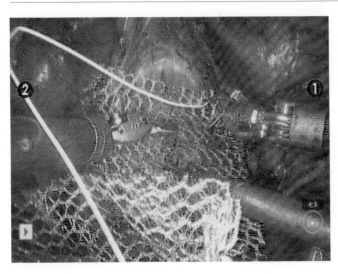 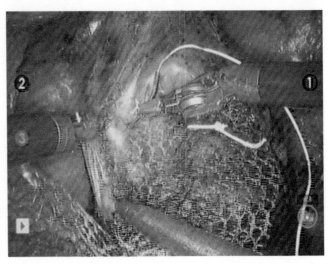

Figure 6-4 The Y-shaped polypropylene mesh graft is first sutured to the anterior vaginal wall, starting at the distal corners. The bladder is retracted cephalad by the fourth arm.

series of interrupted stitches toward the vaginal apex is the most efficient sequence (Figure 6-5). Knots are tied using two surgeon's knots, followed by two half hitches. An attempt is made to achieve healthy bites through the vaginal muscularis without perforating the epithelium.

8. After adequately securing the anterior mesh arm, the vagina is deviated anteriorly and the posterior mesh arm is draped over the posterior vaginal wall with the assistance of the fourth robotic arm, which can hold upward traction on the sacral end of the mesh graft. Starting at the vaginal apex, six to eight interrupted sutures are placed to secure the mesh to the posterior vaginal wall (Figure 6-6). **(See Video 6-4, "Attachment of Posterior Mesh."**) If necessary, the 0-degree scope can be exchanged for a 30-degree up-scope to visualize fully the rectovaginal space.

9. The vaginal EEA sizer is retracted back to allow for the retrieval of the sacral arm of the mesh through the retroperitoneal tunnel. **(See Video 6-5, "Attachment of Mesh to the Promontory."**) The vagina is then deviated toward the sacrum. To ensure that no excessive tension exists, the sacral portion of the mesh graft is sutured to the anterior longitudinal ligament at the promontory using two or three interrupted sutures (Figure 6-7). When placing the needle during this critical juncture, rotating through the ligament along the curvature of the needle is important, as opposed to driving the needle forward and potentially exiting further laterally than expected. Because of the slight traction that exists on the mesh, a slip-knot is preferred over a surgeon's knot. Care is taken to visualize the middle sacral artery and either suture around it or cauterize it. If bleeding is encountered in this space, then a Ray-Tec sponge can be introduced through the accessory port for manual compression. If bleeding continues, then the use of Floseal is recommended for controlling hemostasis.

10. In an attempt to decrease the chance of postoperative bowel obstruction, the mesh is extraperitonealized using a 2-0 Vicryl suture cut to 8-10 inches. Accomplishing this task is easiest by starting at the vaginal apex with a suture similar to a purse-string stitch from the right anterior peritoneum to the right side of the cul-de-sac, coming over the mesh to pick up the left side of the incised peritoneum and then coming back through the left side of the bladder flap (Figure 6-8). After tying down the knot, the vaginal apex is covered. The smaller sacral peritoneal window is easily sutured over the mesh by continuing with a running stitch toward the sacral promontory. Suturing toward the camera and operative instruments, as opposed to away from them, is always easiest; this is especially true during this potentially challenging portion of the procedure.

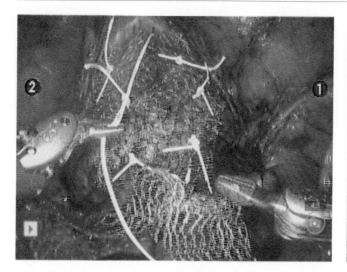

Figure 6-5 The anterior mesh attachment is completed using six sutures of 2-0 Gore-Tex.

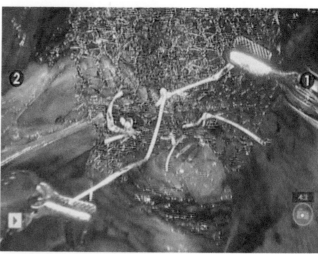

Figure 6-6 Attachment of the posterior arm of the mesh is demonstrated. Upward traction on the sacral portion of the mesh graft is provided by the fourth arm.

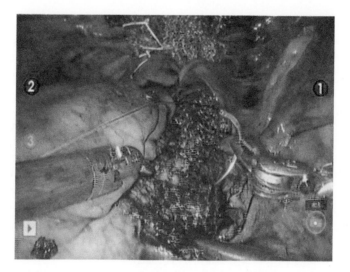

Figure 6-7 Mesh is directly sutured to the anterior longitudinal ligament using two or three stitches and secured with slip knots. Care is taken to avoid undue tension on the mesh graft.

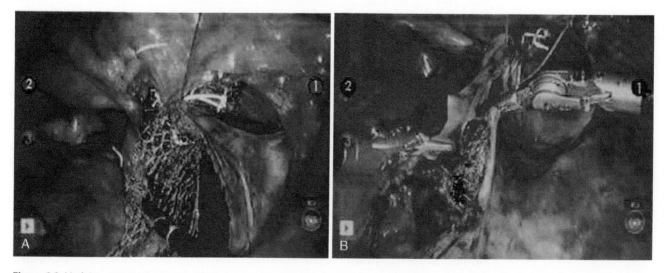

Figure 6-8 Mesh is extraperitonealized by closing the peritoneum from the apex of the vagina with a suture similar to a purse-string stitch, which is then continued to the promontory in a running fashion.

Case 2: Cervicosacropexy

A 45-year-old woman is complaining of pelvic heaviness and a feeling that her "vagina is falling out." She cannot run comfortably as a result of these symptoms. In addition, she has heavy menses and cannot retain a tampon. She also complains of urinary incontinence with physical activity and notes some pain with sexual intercourse. She denies any defecatory dysfunction. An examination reveals stage II-C prolapse with bilateral paravaginal defects and a 10-week size fibroid uterus. When the apex of the vagina is reduced with large cotton swabs, the anterior wall prolapse is reduced. She has a gaping genital hiatus but no posterior wall defects. Urodynamic testing reveals stress urinary incontinence with normal bladder capacity and no voiding dysfunction. Her Papanicolaou test (Pap smear) and endometrial biopsy are benign. Considering her young age, level of physical activity, and completion of childbearing, robotic supracervical hysterectomy, cervicosacropexy, and midurethral sling with a concomitant perineoplasty are recommended. She is advised that leaving the cervix in situ may reduce the chance of mesh erosion and provide an excellent platform for mesh attachment.

Modifications for Cervicosacropexy

1. As in a sacrocolpopexy procedure, the procedure starts at the sacral promontory and first exposes the anterior longitudinal ligament. If the most challenging portion of the procedure cannot be accomplished first, then significant time is not wasted on the completion of all the other steps through a robotic approach.

2. In the event of an intact uterus and benign cervical cytologic results, a supracervical hysterectomy is performed before the steps previously outlined. Leaving the cervix in situ may reduce the chance of mesh erosion, and it provides an excellent platform for mesh attachment. Fully dissecting the anterior and posterior vaginal walls before cervical amputation is easiest, because the upward traction on the corpus improves the visualization of the surgical planes. Once the cervix is amputated, effective vaginal manipulation can present a surgical challenge. Some surgeons use a tenaculum attached to the fourth arm to apply traction on the cervix, but this approach then eliminates this arm for other necessary tasks. Malleable or Breisky-Navratil retractors can be used to delineate the anterior and posterior vaginal fornices but are not always satisfactory, especially if an assistant is not seated between the patient's legs. The Colpo-Probe vaginal fornix delineator (CooperSurgical, Inc., Trumbull, Connecticut) is a useful and inexpensive instrument (Figure 6-9); it not only assists in dissecting the vagina from the bladder and rectum, but it also provides a stable surface during mesh attachment.

3. Cervical amputation should take place below the level of the internal cervical os. The authors of this text do not find it necessary to oversew the cervix; however, hemostasis must be ensured before attaching the mesh.

4. The attachment of the mesh arms to the anterior and posterior vaginal walls and cervix occurs in exactly the same sequence as described for sacrocolpopexy.

Figure 6-9 Colpo-Probe vaginal fornix delineator determines the anterior and posterior vaginal fornices and provides a stable platform against which to suture the mesh graft.

(Courtesy of CooperSurgical, Inc., Trumbull, Connecticut.)

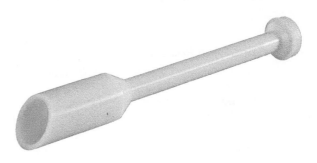

Outcomes

The studies that have evaluated the success of the robotic-assisted sacrocolpopexy have been limited in sample size and mean time follow-up. The largest comparative study of open versus robotic-assisted sacrocolpopexy included 178 patients (73 robotic, 105 abdominal) with a follow-up of only 6 weeks after surgery. (Moreno Sierra et al, 2011) Anatomic outcomes were not significantly different. The robotic approach was associated with less blood loss (103 ml ± 96 ml versus 255 ml ± 155 ml, p <0.001), longer total surgical time (328 minutes ± 55 minutes versus 225 minutes ± 61 minutes, p <0.001), shorter length of hospital stay (1.3 days ± 0.8 days versus 2.7 days ± 1.4 days, p <0.001), and a higher incidence of postoperative fever (4.1% versus 0%, p = 0.04). An evaluation of outcomes 1 year after surgery in 28 patients reported a significant improvement in pelvic floor function over preoperative baseline: the Pelvic Floor Distress Inventory (PFDI-20) (117 versus 38, p <0.001), the Pelvic Floor Impact Questionnaire (PFIQ-7) (60 versus 10, p = 0.001), with stable high sexual function; the Pelvic Organ Prolapse/ Urinary Incontinence Sexual Questionnaire–short version (PISQ-12) (34 versus 36, p = 0.17), and improved pelvic support on the Pelvic Organ Prolapse Quantification (POPQ) system: Point Ba (+3 versus −2, p = 0.001), Point Bp (+0.5 versus −1, p = 0.092), Point C (+2.25 versus −8, p = 0.001). Anatomic cure for vault prolapse was 100% at 1 year. Two mesh exposures occurred, and two subsequent prolapse surgeries were performed to correct distal defects. (Geller, Parnell, Dunivan, 2011) Similarly, in a prospective evaluation of 31 women at 24 months postprocedure, no apical failures were recorded, but quality-of-life outcomes were not measured. (Moreno Sierra, Ortiz Oshiro, Fernandez Perez, 2011) All published studies to date have found that robotic sacrocolpopexy is successful in the treatment of pelvic organ prolapse with a decreased hospital stay, low complication rate, and low morbidity. Each study, however, concluded that more long-term data are required to prove this procedure to be a durable repair. (Geller et al, 2008; Elliott et al, 2004) A recent randomized trial of laparoscopic versus robotic sacrocolpopexy reported significantly longer surgical times and increased postoperative pain in the robotic group, compared with the laparoscopic group. (Paraiso et al, 2011) This trial was conducted in a center renowned for laparoscopic expertise, and total surgical times were notably longer than other published series. (Sullivan, Longaker, Lee, 2001; Summers et al, 2006) The steps previously outlined are designed to improve robotic operative efficiency.

SUMMARY: The da Vinci surgical system facilitates the completion of a colposacropexy or cervicosacropexy in an identical manner performed in an open technique by surgeons who may not possess advanced laparoscopic skills. Full knowledge of the relevant anatomy is critical; significant morbidity can be encountered during the operation if incorrect surgical planes are created. Key points that must be considered during the procedure include the availability of two proficient bedside assistants (typically positioned between the patient's legs and on the right side of the patient), the use of the steep Trendelenburg position to remove the bowels from the surgical field, the correct identification of the sacral promontory, the wide mobilization of the peritoneum, individually fashioned Y-shaped grafts, and the closure of the peritoneum from the vaginal apex toward the sacral promontory. Adequate spacing between the robotic arms is essential to avoid interference between the instruments during the procedure.

Suggested Readings

Akl MN, Long JB, Giles DL, et al: Robotic-assisted sacrocolpopexy: technique and learning curve, *Surg Endosc* 23(10):2390–2394, 2009.

Cosson M, Rajabally R, Bogaert E, et al: Laparoscopic sacrocolpopexy, hysterectomy, and burch colposuspension: feasibility and short-term complications of 77 procedures, *JSLS* 6(2):115–119, 2002.

Culligan PJ, Murphy M, Blackwell L, et al: Long-term success of abdominal sacral colpopexy using synthetic mesh, *Am J Obstet Gynecol* 187(6):1473–1480; discussion 1481–1482, 2002.

Elliott DS, Frank I, Dimarco DS, et al: Gynecologic use of robotically assisted laparoscopy: Sacrocolpopexy for the treatment of high-grade vaginal vault prolapse, *Am J Surg* 188(4A Suppl):52S–56S, 2004.

Elliott DS, Krambeck AE, Chow GK: Long-term results of robotic assisted laparoscopic sacrocolpopexy for the treatment of high grade vaginal vault prolapse, *J Urol* 176(2):655–659, 2006.

Geller EJ, Siddiqui NY, Wu JM, et al: Short-term outcomes of robotic sacrocolpopexy compared with abdominal sacrocolpopexy, *Obstet Gynecol* 112(6):1201–1206, 2008.

Geller EJ, Parnell BA, Dunivan GC: Pelvic floor function before and after robotic sacrocolpopexy: one-year outcomes, *J Minim Invasive Gynecol* 18(3):322–327, 2011.

Maher C, Baessler K, Glazener CM, et al: Surgical management of pelvic organ prolapse in women, *Cochrane Database Syst Rev* (3):CD004014, 2007.

Moreno Sierra J, Ortiz Oshiro E, Fernandez Pérez C, et al: Long-term outcomes after robotic sacrocolpopexy in pelvic organ prolapse: prospective analysis, *Urol Int* 86(4):414–418, 2011.

Nezhat CH, Nezhat F, Nezhat C: Laparoscopic sacral colpopexy for vaginal vault prolapse, *Obstet Gynecol* 84(5):885–888, 1994.

Nygaard IE, McCreery R, Brubaker L, et al: Abdominal sacrocolpopexy: a comprehensive review, *Obstet Gynecol* 104(4):805–823, 2004.

Paraiso MF, Jelovsek JE, Frick A, et al: Laparoscopic compared with robotic sacrocolpopexy for vaginal prolapse: a randomized controlled trial, *Obstet Gynecol* 118(5):1005–1013, 2011.

Ross JW: Techniques of laparoscopic repair of total vault eversion after hysterectomy, *J Am Assoc Gynecol Laparosc* 4(2):173–183, 1997.

Sullivan ES, Longaker CJ, Lee PY: Total pelvic mesh repair: a ten-year experience, *Dis Colon Rectum* 44(6):857–863, 2001.

Summers A, Winkel LA, Hussain HK, et al: The relationship between anterior and apical compartment support, *Am J Obstet Gynecol* 194(5):1438–1443, 2006.

Surgical Management of Apical Vaginal Wall Prolapse

7

Christopher F. Maher MD and Mickey Karram MD

 Video Clips online

7-1 Laparoscopic Trocar Placement Used for Reconstructive Surgical Procedures
7-2 Laparoscopic Adhesiolysis before Laparoscopic Colpopexy
7-3 Laparoscopic Sacral Colpopexy
7-4 Laparoscopic Colposuspension
7-5 Sacrospinous Colpopexy with Anterior Mesh Placement and Posterior Repair
7-6 Techniques to Test for Occult Stress Incontinence
7-7 Total Vaginal Mesh Procedure

7-8 High Uterosacral Vaginal Vault Suspension Performed after Vaginal Hysterectomy
7-9 High Uterosacral Vaginal Vault Suspension for Posthysterectomy Prolapse
7-10 High Intraperitoneal Vaginal Vault Suspension—Revisiting this Pelvic Anatomy
7-11 Laparoscopic Release of Vaginal Scarring before Laparoscopic Colpopexy

Introduction

The incidence of posthysterectomy vaginal wall prolapse that requires surgery has been estimated at 1.3 per 1000 women-years. It remains unclear what proportion of the original hysterectomies in large demographic studies were for prolapse; however, in two randomized trials on the surgical management of vault prolapse conducted by the authors of this text, two thirds of the women underwent hysterectomies for prior prolapse. The figures from these trials are supported by data suggesting that the risk of prolapse surgery is 4.7 times higher in women whose initial hysterectomy was to correct prolapse and 8 times higher if preoperative prolapse stage II or higher was present. As a result of its recurrent nature, vault prolapse remains a challenging problem for both the patient and the surgeon.

This chapter reviews the indications and techniques used to perform a variety of procedures that have been successful in supporting the prolapsed vaginal apex.

Background

In reviewing the literature, the abdominal sacral colpopexy (ASC) remains the "gold standard" in the management of vault prolapse. (Nygaard et al, 2004; Maher et al, 2007) The Cochrane review noted three randomized controlled trials (RCTs), in which the ASC was associated with a lower rate of recurrent vault prolapse and less dyspareunia, as compared with sacrospinous colpopexy. However, the abdominal approach was also associated with longer surgical time and admission time, greater blood loss, and a slower return to performing activities of daily living.

The uterosacral vault suspension remains a popular vaginal option. In a recent metaanalysis, Margulies and colleagues (2010) reviewed over 800 uterosacral cases and found the success rates for anterior, apical, and posterior compartments were 81%,

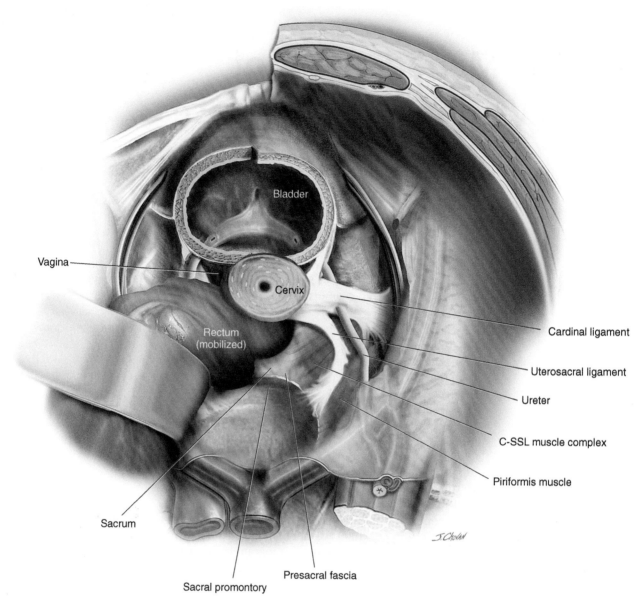

Figure 7-1 The anatomy of the support structures of the uterus and upper vagina is demonstrated. The relationship among the uterosacral ligament, the ureter, the coccygeus–sacrospinous ligament (C-SSL) muscle complex, and the presacral fascia is noted.

(From Baggish MS, Karram MM: Atlas of pelvic anatomy and gynecologic surgery, ed 3, St Louis, 2011, Elsevier.)

98%, and 87%, respectively. They also reported that associated preoperative stage III anterior compartment prolapse was associated with a significantly higher failure rate than stage II anterior compartment prolapse. Ureteric obstruction was the most common complication and was reported in 15 patients (1.8%). Figure 7-1 demonstrates the relationship among the uterosacral ligament, the ureter, the coccygeus–sacrospinous ligament (C-SSL) muscle complex, and the presacral fascia. In 10 patients, the removal of the offending uterosacral suspension suture relieved the obstruction, and ureteral reimplantation was required in 5 patients (0.6%). Blood transfusion was reported in 11 patients (1.3%). Intraoperative complications were low and included a cystotomy during hysterectomy (0.1%), and 2 patients had bowel injuries (0.2%). (Margulies, Rogers, Morgan, 2010) In a recent RCT, Rondini and associates compared open sacral colpopexy (n = 54) and high uterosacral ligament vault suspension (HUSLS) (n = 56) and demonstrated similar findings to the sacrospinous colpopexy previously reported.

Higher objective success rates and lower rates of recurrences were reported in the anterior and posterior compartments. Although the reoperation rate for prolapse was significantly lower after sacral colpopexy (5% as compared with 17.8% in the uterosacral suspension group), both intraoperative complications (3.7% versus 0%, p = 0.15) and postoperative complications (20.4% versus 7.3%, p = 0.047) were higher after the sacral colpopexy, as compared with HUSLS.

After the uterosacral ligament suspension (USLS) and sacrospinous colpopexy, recurrent anterior compartment prolapse remains the most common site of failure. With this in mind, when vaginally performing apical prolapse surgery, some surgeons are now incorporating anterior compartment mesh with sacrospinous colpopexy and uterosacral suspensions; however, little data on the efficacy of this approach are available at this stage. Obliterative procedures are also an option in the older patient who is not sexually active. (See Chapter 10 for a detailed discussion of the procedures.)

In an attempt to decrease the perioperative morbidity associated with open sacral colpopexy, the laparoscopic sacral colpopexy (LSC) (Higgs, Chua, Smith, 2005; Paraiso et al, 2005; Klauschie et al, 2009; North et al, 2009), the robotic sacral colpopexy (Paraiso et al, 2011), and the vaginal mesh procedures (VMPs) (Fatton et al, 2007; Caquant et al, 2008) have increased in popularity. A recently completed RCT, in which the LSC and the total vaginal mesh (TVM) technique were compared with a 2-year follow-up, demonstrated a significantly higher anatomic success rate (LSC at 77% versus TVM at 43%), higher patient satisfaction (87 patients for LSC versus 79 patients for TVM,) longer total vaginal length (TVL) (LSC at 8.83 cm versus TVM at 7.81 cm), and significantly lower reoperation rate after the LSC, as compared with TVM (5% versus 22%, respectively). (Maher et al, 2011) The high reoperation rate after VMPs was also reported by Diwadkar and associates (2009) who systematically examined the complication and reoperation rates after traditional vaginal surgery, sacrocolpopexy, and vaginal mesh kit procedures. Complications were classified using the Clavien-Dindo grading system—grade IIIa (intervention not requiring general anesthesia) and grade IIIb (intervention under general anesthesia) rates were highest in the mesh kit group as a result of higher rates of mesh erosion (198 of 3425) and fistulae (8 of 3425). Reoperation rates for prolapse recurrence were highest in the traditional vaginal surgery group (308 of 7827). The total reoperation rate was greatest in the mesh kit group (291 of 3425, 8.5%). (Diwadkar et al, 2009)

The shorter TVL after the TVM procedure, as compared with LSC and reported in one prospective RCT (Maher et al, 2011), has also been reported in a multicenter retrospective chart review; this review compared Prolift VMP (206 patients), USLS (231 patients), and ASC (305 patients). No difference in apical success after VMP (98.8%) was demonstrated, compared with USLS (99.1%) or ASC (99.3%); however, the average elevation of the vaginal apex was lower after VMP (–6.9 cm) than USLS (–8.05 cm) and ASC (–8.5 cm) (both p = 0.001). (Sanses et al, 2009) In contrast, a recently prospective case series of 46 women with vault prolapse at 12 months reported excellent outcomes with a 91% overall objective success rate, a mesh erosion rate of 15% with the TVL decreasing from 8.8 to 8.5 cm postoperatively. (Milani, Withagen, Vierhout, 2009) Recently, Iglesia and colleagues (2010) reported a double blind RCT comparing Prolift (33 patients) and uterosacral native repair (32 patients) for vaginal prolapse. They found at 10 months the recurrence rate was 59% in the mesh group, as compared with 70% in the nonmesh group (p = 0.28). Unfortunately, the study was terminated early because a predetermined review board mesh erosion rate of 15% was surpassed. The authors questioned the value of polypropylene mesh grafts in prolapse surgery. More recently, Withagen and associates (2011) compared native tissue repairs in 97 women with Prolift mesh repairs in 93 women, all of whom underwent prior prolapse surgery. At 1 year, the authors reported the recurrence rate in the treated compartment was 45.2% in the conventional (nonmesh) group, as compared with 9.6% in the mesh group (p <0.001; odds ratio [OR], 7.7, 95% CI 3.3 to 18. No differences in subjective assessment and patient satisfaction were identified, and the mesh extrusion rate was 17%. On closer evaluation, this study failed to control selection and reporting bias and to report a meaningful definition of the objective assessment. Preoperatively, the nonmesh group is significantly different from the mesh group on a number of important preoperative assessments, and readers should be cautious when drawing conclusions from this trial. Unfortunately, 7 years after commercial mesh kits have been introduced into the market, no definitive level-one evidence confirms that these interventions are superior to the native tissue repairs in the management of apical prolapse.

In July 2011, the U.S. Food and Drug Administration (FDA) released a transvaginal mesh alert after an increased number of adverse events were reported; (the full document is available at http://www.fda.gov/MedicalDevices/Safety/AlertsandNotices/ ucm262435.htm). Mesh erosions account for 38% of these alerts and occur in an estimated 10% of patients with over one half requiring at least one surgical intervention to address the erosion. Interestingly, vaginal pain and dyspareunia, together, account for the greatest number of reports (39%) and remain poorly characterized and reported in the literature. After conducting an extensive literature review, the FDA came to the following conclusions relevant to the apical compartment:

1. Mesh augmentation for transvaginal apical or posterior repair does not appear to provide any added benefit, compared with traditional native tissue suture repair.

2. Mesh abdominally placed for pelvic organ prolapse (POP) repair may result in less recurrent prolapse and, when compared with transvaginal meshes, appears to have lower complication rates.

The FDA also suggested that clinicians adhere to the following recommendations:

1. Recognize that, in most cases, POP can be successfully treated without mesh, thus avoiding the risk of mesh-related complications. Mesh surgery should only be performed after weighing the risks and benefits of surgery with mesh versus all surgical and nonsurgical alternatives.

2. The following factors should be considered before placing surgical mesh:

   - Surgical mesh is a permanent implant that may make future surgical repair more challenging.

   - Mesh procedures may place the patient at risk for requiring additional surgery for the development of new complications.

   - Removal of mesh as a result of mesh complications may involve multiple surgeries and significantly impair the patient's quality of life. Complete removal of mesh may not be possible and may not result in the complete resolution of complications, including pain.

   - Mesh abdominally placed for POP repair may result in lower rates of mesh complications, compared with transvaginal POP surgery with mesh.

3. Inform the patient about the benefits and risks of nonsurgical options, nonmesh surgery, surgical mesh abdominally placed, and the likely success of these alternatives, compared with transvaginal surgery with mesh.

4. Notify the patient if mesh will be used in her POP surgery, and provide the patient with information about the specific product used.

5. Ensure that the patient understands the postoperative risks and complications of mesh surgery, as well as the limited long-term outcomes data.

Finally, as of this writing and in a preliminary report due to be released after September 2012, the FDA advisory meeting concluded the following:

- The safety of transvaginal meshes has not been established.

- Depending on the compartment, the efficacy of transvaginal meshes has not been established to be more effective than traditional repairs.

- Safety and efficacy of mesh at sacral colpopexy has been established.

Currently, most ASCs can be endoscopically performed. The robotic approach to the sacral colpopexy is discussed fully in Chapter 6; however, in a recent RCT in which robotic and laparoscopic approaches were compared, Paraiso and colleagues (2011) reported that the robotic procedure was associated with longer surgical time, longer postoperative use of nonsteroidal pain medications, and was more expensive than the

Table 7-1 Advantages and Disadvantages of Different Approaches to Sacral Colpopexy

	Open	Laparoscopic	Robotic
Evaluation	Significant	Limited	Limited
Skills required	Competent pelvic surgeon with decreased colposuspension and hysterectomy rates. Reduction in open abdominal skills	Competent laparoscopic surgical suturing and dissection skills	Competent robot learning curve. Easier to master suturing skills than laparoscopic approach. Greater precision sutures
Technical considerations	Potentially challenging. Clearly achievable	Carbon dioxide insufflation, providing excellent exposure, vision, and access during dissection. Everyone OT see surgery = transparency	Carbon dioxide insufflation, providing excellent exposure and access, especially dissection vision. Increased three-dimensional visualization. Everyone OT see surgery = transparency
Tactile feedback	Excellent aids in dissection	Excellent aids in dissection	No tactile feedback, potentially increasing risk for viscus injury
Adhesions	Achievable	Achievable	Problematic
Surgical time	Equal	Equal	Increased
Admission time	Increased	Reduced	Reduced
Success rates	Equivalent	Equivalent	Little data are available
Cost	Standard	Maybe reduced	Increased
Ergonomic factors	Equal	Equal	Improved

laparoscopic approach. At 1 year, no differences in anatomic and functional outcomes have been reported, although the study was significantly underpowered to detect any differences in these outcomes; further evaluation of both laparoscopic and robotic approaches is required. Table 7-1 compares the advantages and disadvantages of the open, laparoscopic, and robotic sacral colpopexy.

When isolated, mild apical (descent to midpoint vagina) requires surgery vaginal hysterectomy with culdoplasty (see Chapter 4) or vaginal enterocele repair (see chapter 9) is usually sufficient to provide a vagina of adequate length. As more of the anterior and or posterior vaginal walls are everted, the more complex the repair becomes. Usually, a more formal apical repair in conjunction with a repair of the anterior and/or posterior vaginal wall is required (Figure 7-2). The goal of any apical suspension should be to provide a high durable suspension of the apex without creating a significant distortion to the vaginal axis. In general, if the apex can be suspended to the level of the ischial spine, then the vaginal length will be approximately 9 cm.

A variety of vault suspending surgeries are presented and discussed in the following case presentations and accompanying videos. The reader should recognize that every case must be individualized; no single surgical procedure is likely to be successful for all patients. The pelvic floor surgeon should be capable of performing a variety of procedures to meet the specific needs of every patient. Furthermore, every surgeon should continually monitor the literature and audit their own conclusions to ensure the best possible outcomes for patients.

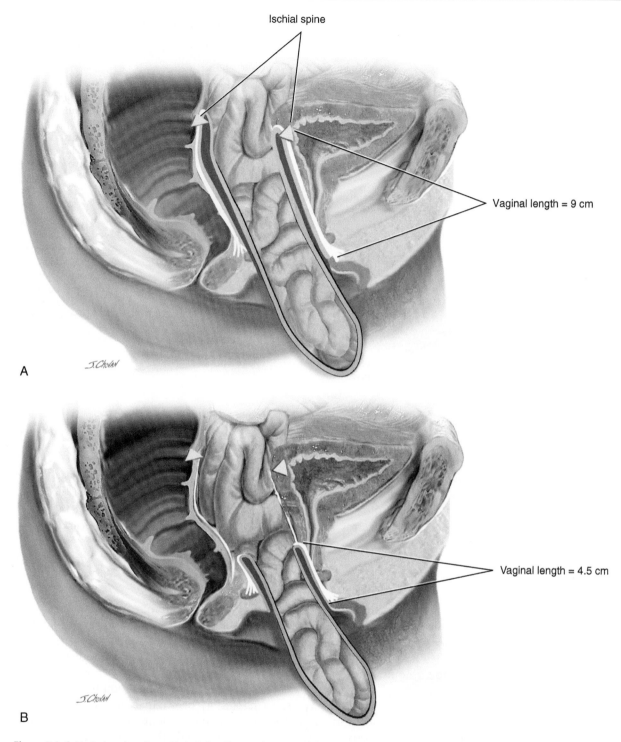

Figure 7-2 A, Vaginal vault prolapsed in isolation. The good support of the anterior and posterior vaginal walls is noted. Such a situation simply requires the excision of the enterocele sac and the closure of the defect at the level of the bladder neck, which will support the apex of the vagina, maintaining adequate vaginal length. **B,** Approximately 50% of the length of the anterior and posterior vaginal walls is everted. Such a situation requires the suspension of the apex to the level of the ischial spine, in conjunction with the restoration of support of the upper portion of the anterior and posterior vaginal walls.

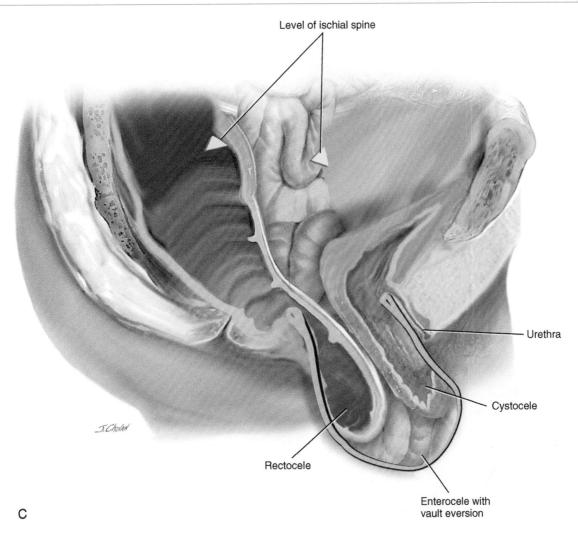

Level of ischial spine

Urethra

Cystocele

Rectocele

Enterocele with
vault eversion

C

Figure 7-2, cont'd. C, Complete vaginal vault prolapse with complete eversion of the anterior and posterior vaginal walls is demonstrated. Such a situation requires a more complex repair; the prolapsed vaginal vault needs to be suspended high up into the pelvic cavity to the level of the ischial spines, which must be achieved in conjunction with other procedures that need to be performed to provide durable support to the anterior and posterior vaginal walls.

(From Baggish MS, Karram MM: Atlas of pelvic anatomy and gynecologic surgery, *ed 3, St Louis, 2011, Elsevier.)*

Case 1: Laparoscopic Sacral Colpopexy

A 56-year-old patient has posthysterectomy vaginal vault prolapse and urinary incontinence. Her previous surgeries included vaginal hysterectomy and repair and an appendectomy. An examination confirms anterior compartment at the introitus and the vault extending 3 cm beyond the introitus. Urodynamic testing demonstrates a stable bladder and significant urinary stress incontinence with no voiding dysfunction. This patient consents to an LSC and colposuspension (Figures 7-3, 7-4, and 7-5). Figure 7-6 shows a sagittal view.

Surgical Steps: Laparoscopic Sacral Colpopexy

1. Trocar placement: Figure 7-7 illustrates the anterior abdominal wall vasculature and preferred trocar placement. A 10-mm re-useable Hassan trocar is placed subumbilically under direct vision. Secondary trocars are introduced under laparoscopic vision with three further trocars used:

   a. 10-mm trocar: Is placed left of the iliac fossa approximately 2 cm medial and superior to the anterosuperior iliac crest for the skin incision, and entry in the abdomen is lateral to the inferior epigastric vessels. This trocar is used to introduce mesh and needles. Alternatively, a 5-mm

Figure 7-3 Laparoscopic view of anterior abdominal wall architecture; medial umbilical ligament* inferior epigastric vessel ** and correct entry point of trocar lateral to inferior epigastric vessel ***.

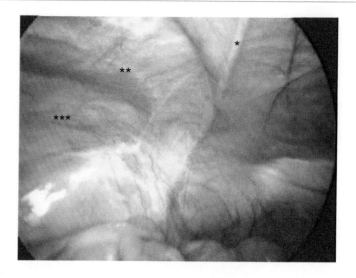

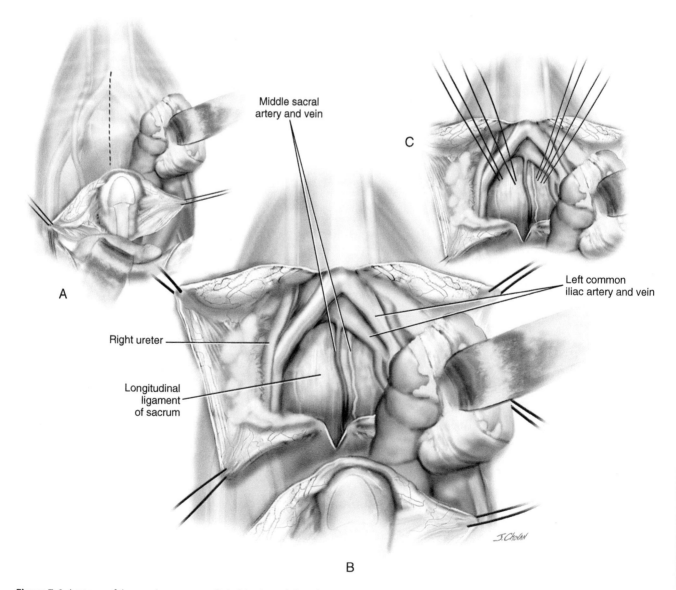

Figure 7-4 Anatomy of the sacral promontory. **A,** Incision is made into the peritoneum. **B,** Dissection of the longitudinal ligament of the promontory is demonstrated. The vascularity of this area is noted. **C,** Permanent sutures are placed through the longitudinal ligament of the sacrum.

(From Baggish MS, Karram MM: Atlas of pelvic anatomy and gynecologic surgery, ed 3, St Louis, 2011, Elsevier.)

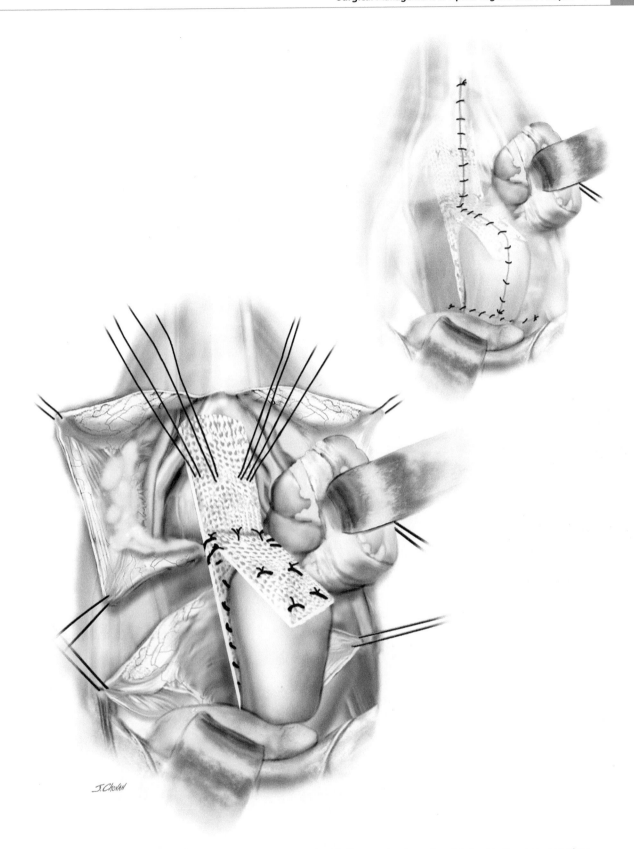

Figure 7-5 The mesh is attached to the sacrum using two pieces of mesh. The anterior piece of mesh is fixed to the upper part of the anterior posterior vaginal wall and extends much farther down. Both pieces are brought together and fixed to the sacral promontory. Closure of the peritoneum over the mesh is shown *(inset)*.

(From Baggish MS, Karram MM: Atlas of pelvic anatomy and gynecologic surgery, ed 3, St Louis, 2011, Elsevier.)

Figure 7-6 A second piece of mesh is attached to the upper part of anterior vaginal wall and sewn to a posterior piece of the mesh.

(From Baggish MS, Karram MM: Atlas of pelvic anatomy and gynecologic surgery, ed 3, St Louis, 2011, Elsevier.)

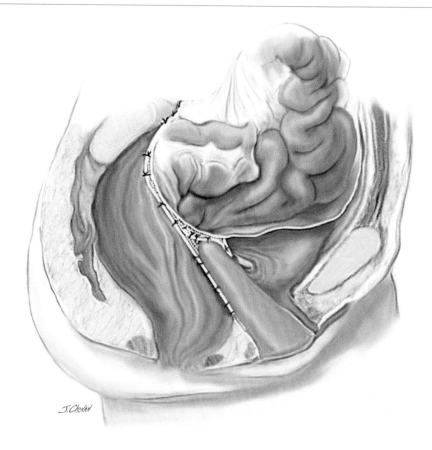

Figure 7-7 Sutures have been appropriately placed on each side of the proximal urethral and bladder neck. The figure-of-8 bites are taken through the vagina. Double-armed sutures are used to ensure that the end of each suture can be brought up through the ipsilateral Cooper ligament, thus allowing the sutures to be tied above the ligament.

(From Baggish MS, Karram MM: Atlas of pelvic anatomy and gynecologic surgery, ed 3, St Louis, 2011, Elsevier.)

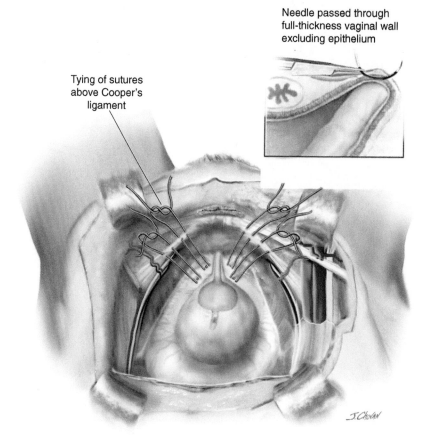

Needle passed through full-thickness vaginal wall excluding epithelium

Tying of sutures above Cooper's ligament

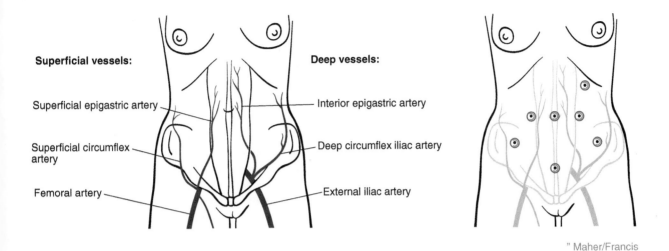

Coronal View A
Anterior abdominal wall vasculature

Superficial vessels:

Superficial epigastric artery

Superficial circumflex artery

Femoral artery

Coronal View B
Primary and secondary trocar site placements

Deep vessels:

Interior epigastric artery

Deep circumflex iliac artery

External iliac artery

" Maher/Francis

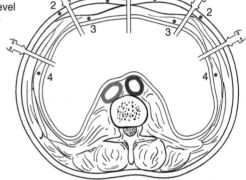

Transverse view
just below the level
of the umbilicus

1 Superficial epigastric artery
2 Superficial circumflex iliac artery
3 Interior epigastric artery
4 Deep circumflex iliac artery

Figure 7-8 The relationship of the anterior abdominal wall vasculature is demonstrated in coronal and transverse views. The suggested trocar placement is visualized.

with a high postvoid and needles being introduced through the umbilical incision with the camera removed.

b. 5-mm trocar is placed 6 cm left of umbilicus and entry under vision is lateral to inferior of the epigastric vessels (see Figure 7-8). (**See Video 7-1, "Laparoscopic Trocar Placement Used for Reconstructive Surgical Procedures"** 🎥 for a demonstration of laparoscopic trocar placement.)

c. 5-mm trocar in right iliac fossa with identical landmarks to lower left trocar above.

2. Figure 7-7 highlights the common trocar positions in relation to the anterior abdominal wall vessels. In patients with a prior vertical midline incision, a Palmer's point entry technique can be used to minimize the risk of bowel perforation entry. (**See Video 7-1** 🎥 for a demonstration of the laparoscopic entry technique.)

3. Steep Trendelenburg position facilitates the emptying of the small and large bowels from the pelvis.

4. Any adhesions present should be mobilized; significant adhesiolysis, defined as greater than 45 minutes, occurs in 25% of posthysterectomy cases. (**See Video 7-2, "Laparoscopic**

Adhesiolysis before Laparoscopic Colpopexy," 📹 for a video demonstration of laparoscopic adhesiolysis in three patients undergoing laparoscopy sacral colpopexy.)

5. The peritoneum is opened from the sacral promontory to the vault with unipolar scissors, staying medial to the uterosacral ligament and lateral to the large bowel. The scissors are in the left upper trocar, and nontraumatic forceps retract the peritoneum from the left and right lower trocars.

6. Once the dissection is at the vault, a nonheat and energy-conducting Apple vaginal probe is introduced into the vagina. The probe features blunt polymer tips for atraumatic use, surgical-grade stainless steel shafts, and color-coded anodized aluminum handles; it offers counter traction that facilitates the dissection of the bladder and bowel from the vagina.

7. For anterior dissection, atraumatic forceps in the left lower trocar reflects the bladder, and sharp dissection of the bladder from the vagina is performed with scissors in the left upper trocar. The dissection continues centrally to the level of the trigone, which is identified when the bladder will no longer mobilize from the vagina at approximately 7 cm along the anterior wall dissection.

8. Rectovaginal space is created with the vaginal probe acutely anteverted and atraumatic forceps in the left lower trocar, reflecting the bowel inferiorly, and let upper trocar space to approximately 8 cm along the posterior vaginal wall with the minimal use of electrosurgical energy and dissection.

9. The mesh is prepared as demonstrated in Video 7-3 A 15 × 15 cm sheet of Ultrapro (JJ Ethicon) mesh is cut on the diagonal to create a posterior leaf of mesh approximately 5 to 6 cm wide and 22 cm long. A second anterior leaf is harvested approximately 5 to 6 cm wide and 8 cm long. These are sutured together using interrupted 2.0 polydioxanone suture (PDS).

10. The anterior mesh is secured to the vagina with two to three sutures (2.0 PDS) commencing with distal sutures and working toward the vault. The vaginal is then acutely anteverted, and the posterior leaf is secured to the vagina with two to three sutures (2.0 PDS) commencing distally and working toward the vault.

11. The vaginal probe is removed, and the posterior tail of the mesh is secured to the sacral promontory with nonabsorbable hernia tacks. Excellent exposure of the ligament is required to avoid injury to the surrounding vasculature. The potential advantages of the tacks over sutures are that they are hemostatic and can be easily inserted.

12. The retroperitoneum is closed with a continuous 2.0 PDS to ensure that no mesh is visible intraperitoneally at the completion of the surgery. Using this technique, virtually no bowel obstruction or symptoms of stasis occur, which seem common in some sacral colpopexy series.

13. Steep Trendelenburg position can be reduced, and the retropubic space is then entered if continence or prolapse surgery is to be performed.

14. Cystoscopic examination is performed to ensure that the ureters are patent and the bladder mucosa is intact.

15. Posterior colpoperineorrhaphy is usually required to complete the procedure.

16. The indwelling catheter is removed the next morning (6:00 AM), and a trial of void completed.

17. Antibiotics are initiated, thromboembolic stockings are worn for 7 days, and self-administered enoxaparin sodium (Clexane) (20 mg) is injected daily for 5 days for all patients. (**See Video 7-3, "Laparoscopic Sacral Colpopexy"** 📹 and **Video 7-4, "Laparoscopic Colposuspension"** 📹 for demonstrations of LSC and laparoscopic colposuspension.)

Case Discussion

The popularity and excellent results from sacral colpopexy are reported in three RCTs (Benson, 1996; Lo, 1998; Maher et al, 2004); however, significant morbidity, including longer surgical time, longer admission time, and slower return to activities of daily living, has caused many clinicians to consider the laparoscopic approach to this surgery. A comparison of the laparoscopic arm of the authors' 2011 RCT trial with the open sacral colpopexy arm of the 2004 RCT study (Table 7-2) demonstrates a similar surgical time, reduced blood loss, and reduced lengths of time for admission and recovery with similar objective outcomes. Most of this advantage arises from the reduced morbidity associated with the laparoscopic access, as compared with laparotomy. The laparoscopic surgeon needs to be proficient in a variety of laparoscopic entry techniques. (**See Video 7-1,**

Table 7-2 Comparisons of Outcomes from Open and Laparoscopic Sacral Colpopexy

	Open Sacral Colpopexy[a]	Laparoscopic Sacral Colpopexy[b]
Number	46	53
Surgical time (in minutes)	106	97
Blood loss (ml)	362	100
Inpatient days	5.4	2
Days to return to performing ADLs	34	21
Transfusions	One	One
Intraoperative complications	One cystotomy	One cystotomy, one enterotomy
Complications reoperation	Two incisional hernia, one removed mesh, two POP surgeries	One trocar hernia, one mesh erosion, one TVT
Mesh erosions	One	One
Patient satisfaction	85	87
Overall success rate	76%	77%
Length of review	24 months	24 months

ADLs, Activities of daily living; LSC, laparoscopic sacral colpopexy, POP, pelvic organ prolapse; TVT, tension-free vaginal tape.
[a]Maher CF, Qatawneh AM, Dwyer PL, et al: Abdominal sacral colpopexy or vaginal sacrospinous colpopexy for vaginal vault prolapse: a prospective randomized study. *Am J Obstet Gynecol* 190(1):20–26, 2004.
[b]Maher CF, Feiner B, DeCuyper EM, et al: Laparoscopic sacral colpopexy versus total vaginal mesh for the management of vaginal vault prolapse: a randomised controlled trial. *Am J Obstet Gynecol* 204(4):360.e1-e7, 2011.

"Laparoscopic Trocar Placement Used for Reconstructive Surgical Procedures" ⌦ for a video demonstration of laparoscopic entry techniques.) A distinct advantage of the laparoscopic approach relates to improved vision, especially in the posterior compartment, which translates to greater precision in the surgery. The raised intraabdominal pressure from the installation of carbon dioxide and camera magnification also expedite the dissection to create the vesicovaginal and rectovaginal spaces. A final advantage of the laparoscopic approach is improved vision, which hastens the teaching of this procedure for the trainee, eases the supervisory difficulties associated with laparotomy, and improves the accountability of surgery with all members of the surgical team able to monitor the surgical progress. The disadvantage of the LSC is the learning curve associated with intraperitoneal suturing and dissection; however, once these skills are mastered, this procedure is able to be mastered quickly by all competent pelvic floor surgeons. As a result of the recent challenges associated with traditional laparoscopic suturing, many surgeons have chosen to perform ASC robotically (see Chapter 6).

Case 2: Sacrospinous Colpopexy with Anterior Mesh Placement and Posterior Repair

 View: Video 7-5

A 75-year-old patient, who previously underwent a vaginal hysterectomy with anterior and posterior colporrhaphy, now has posthysterectomy vault prolapse extending 5 cm beyond the introitus. With the prolapse-reduced urodynamics demonstrated, no voiding difficulties or occult stress incontinence is revealed. Although this patient would be suitable for a variety of procedures, the authors of this text elected to proceed with a sacrospinous colpopexy with the placement of anterior vaginal mesh and posterior repair.

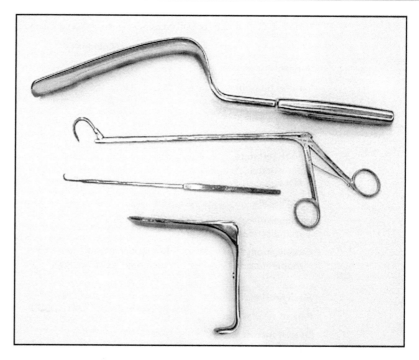

Figure 7-9 Sacrospinous tray *(from top to bottom)*: Breisky-Navratil retractor, Miya hook, nerve hook for retrieving sutures, and notched speculum to facilitate the retrieval of sutures.

Surgical Steps

1. Hydrodissection with 50 ml Marcaine solution 0.25% with adrenalin is injected under the vaginal mucosa.

2. The vaginal mucosa is incised from the posterior fourchette to the external urethral meatus.

3. Using sharp dissection, the bladder, bowel, and/or enterocele are reflected medially. Traction and counter-traction with atraumatic forceps on the viscus and Allis clamps on the vaginal wall tremendously facilitate dissection in the appropriate plane.

4. Anteriorly, after the bladder is centrally mobilized with sharp dissection, the surgeon's finger is introduced beneath the pubic rami to create bilateral obturator paravesical spaces. Posteriorly, once the rectum is medially mobilized, the sacrospinous space is opened medially and proximally to the puborectalis muscle. The sacrospinous ligament, which runs medially from the ischial spine to the lateral aspect of the lower sacrum, is palpated.

5. The Prolift anterior mesh guide is inserted through the obturator space beneath the ischiopubic rami and enters the paravesical space between the fingers of the surgeon's hand. The bladder is protected from puncture by a Breisky-Navratil retractor (Figure 7-9).

6. Two 2.0 PDS are passed 1 cm medial to the ischial spine through the right sacrospinous ligament using the Miya Hook (Figure 7-10).

7. The rectovaginal fascia is plicated with a continuous 2.0 PDS.

8. The first sacrospinous suture is passed through the distal leaf of the Prolift mesh and tied to the right sacrospinous ligament, thus ensuring continuity of support between anterior compartment and vault.

9. The second sacrospinous suture passes through each side of the vaginal mucosa incision to the newly created vault.

10. The vaginal mucosa is closed using continuous 2.0 Vicryl stitches, and the remaining sacrospinous suture is tied.

11. Perineoplasty is performed.

12. A rectal examination is performed to ensure that the rectal mucosa is intact; a cystoscopic examination ensures that the ureters are patent and the bladder is intact.

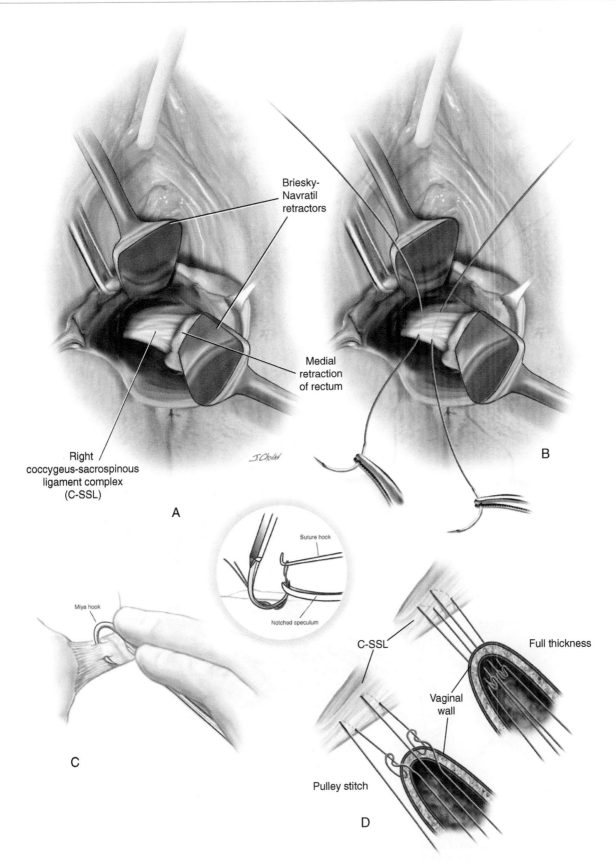

Figure 7-10 A, Exposure of the right sacrospinous ligament is demonstrated. **B,** Suture is passed through the sacrospinous ligament. **C,** Technique of passage of a Miya hook through the ligament is visualized, as well as the technique of retrieval of the suture *(inset).* **D,** Technique of fixing the vaginal apex to the coccygeus–sacrospinous ligament (C-SSL) is demonstrated. If a pulley stitch is performed, then permanent sutures are used. If the sutures are passed through the vaginal epithelium and tied in the vaginal lumen, then delayed absorbable sutures are used.

(Modified from Baggish MS, Karram MM: Atlas of pelvic anatomy and gynecologic surgery, *ed 3, St Louis, 2011, Elsevier.)*

13. Antibiotics are initiated, thromboembolic stockings are worn for 7 days, and self-administered enoxaparin sodium (Clexane) (20 mg) is injected daily for 5 days for every patient. Patients at high risk of thromboembolic events must complete an extended course of self-administered Clexane (40 mg).

14. The vaginal pack is removed at 6:00 AM after surgery, and the indwelling catheter is removed at 12:00 PM the next day and a formal trial of void is commenced.

See Video 7-5, "Sacrospinous Colpopexy with Anterior Mesh Placement and Posterior Repair" for a video demonstration.

Case Discussion

Sacrospinous colpopexy for apical compartment prolapse has been shown to have a lower anatomic success rate than the open ASC with the overwhelming problem remaining the recurrent anterior compartment prolapse. When using the vaginal approach to vault prolapse, the authors of this text nearly always perform this combination of sacrospinous colpopexy, anterior mesh kit with the proximal tail connected to the right sacrospinous colpopexy, and native tissue rectovaginal fascial plication as required and diagrammatically shown in Figure 7-11. The introduction of the

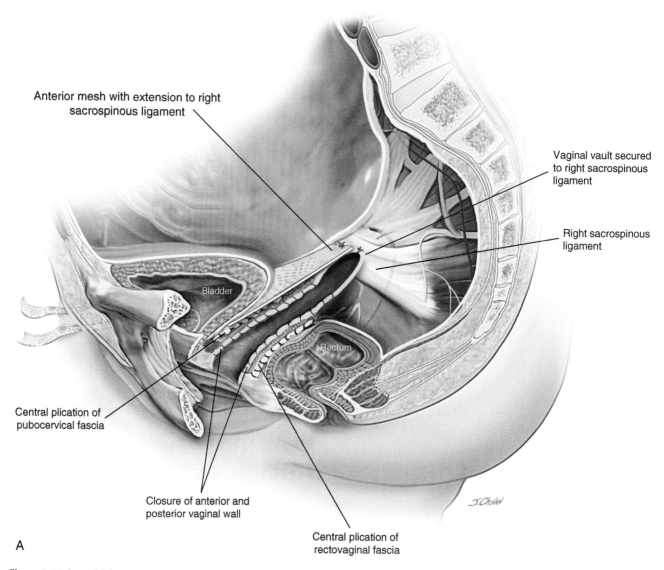

Anterior mesh with extension to right sacrospinous ligament

Vaginal vault secured to right sacrospinous ligament

Right sacrospinous ligament

Bladder

Rectum

Central plication of pubocervical fascia

Closure of anterior and posterior vaginal wall

Central plication of rectovaginal fascia

A

Figure 7-11 Sagittal **(A)** and coronal **(B)** views of the sacrospinous colpopexy, anterior mesh with extension to the sacrospinous ligament, and native tissue posterior repair for vaginal vault prolapsed are visualized.

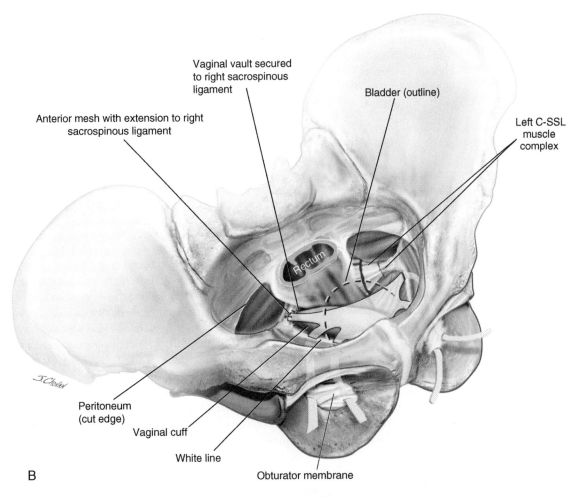

Vaginal vault secured
to right sacrospinous
ligament

Bladder (outline)

Anterior mesh with extension to right
sacrospinous ligament

Left C-SSL
muscle
complex

Rectum

Peritoneum
(cut edge)

Vaginal cuff

White line

Obturator membrane

B

Figure 7-11, cont'd.

anterior mesh has been shown to reduce recurrent anterior compartment prolapse. In addition, the connection of the mesh to the right sacrospinous ligament, which allows a continuous communication between anterior and apical compartments, is attractive and may address the anterior compartment prolapse concerns associated with the traditional sacrospinous colpopexy.

Considering the excellent outcomes of LSC, the authors nearly always choose this approach to correct vault prolapse. Possible indications when the vaginal approach would be favored include the following: (1) gross obesity with a body mass index (BMI) greater than 40, (2) prior pelvic external beam radiation, (3) anterior abdominal wall stomas, (4) extensive prior abdominal surgeries, including adhesiolysis, peritonitis, and bowel resections with protracted recoveries, (5) medically infirm or frail and unable to tolerate general anesthesia or the Trendelenburg position, and (6) patient preference.

Occult stress urinary incontinence, defined as stress incontinence observed only after the reduction of co-existent prolapse (Haylen et al, 2010), is a second issue to be considered. No standardized technique for assessing occult stress incontinence is available. A variety of methods have been described **See Video 7.6, "Techniques to Test for Occult Stress Incontinence"** for prolapse reduction including reducing the prolapse manually with sponge-holding forceps or with ring pessary and with the bladder filled to 300 ml. The issue is currently controversial among clinicians arriving at opposite conclusions after large trials. The incidence of occult stress incontinence in stress continent women undergoing surgery for prolapse varies from 14% to 36%. (Jundt et al, 2010; Maher et al, 2004) The Cochrane review after metaanalysis could not demonstrate a benefit in performing continence surgery at the time of prolapse surgery in those with occult stress incontinence, as compared with not performing continence surgery because of very significant heterogeneity in the data. However, they estimated that 20% of women with occult stress incontinence would benefit from continence surgery being performed at the time of prolapse surgery and recommended, until better data are available, that clinicians discuss these figures with their patients preoperatively. (Maher et al, 2010) The authors of this text have always tended to perform continence surgery at the time of prolapse surgery in women with occult stress incontinence. (See Chapter 3 for a more detailed discussion of evaluating lower urinary tract function in patients with POP.)

Case 3: Total Vaginal Mesh Procedure

 View: Video 7-7

A 72-year-old woman with posthysterectomy vaginal prolapse reports symptoms of voiding dysfunction and recurrent urinary tract infections for the last 2 years. She previously underwent vaginal hysterectomy and repair 15 years earlier and has mild hypertension. A vaginal examination with straining reveals the anterior compartment extending beyond the introitus by 8 cm with the vault 2 cm beyond the introitus and moderate posterior compartment prolapse. Urodynamic tests were performed and demonstrated significant voiding dysfunction with the maximal flow rate of 9 ml/sec and low detrusor voiding pressure of 10 cm H_2O. The residual urine was 400 ml on the first void and 500 ml on a second void. With the prolapse reduced with a ring pessary, the residual urine remained at 450 ml.

Clean intermittent self-catheterization (CISC) is introduced with antibiotics. After a detailed discussion of a variety of options, the patient elects to proceed with a TVM procedure in the hopes of avoiding a second recurrence of her prolapse. The patient is fully aware of the potential future complications related to synthetic mesh placement. She also accepts the likelihood of ongoing voiding dysfunction requiring CISC postoperatively and has signed a procedure-specific consent form. The surgical steps include the following:

1. Hydrodissection with 60 ml Marcaine solution 0.25% with adrenalin is introduced under the vaginal mucosa and into paravesical and pararectal spaces bilaterally.

2. The vaginal mucosa is opened from the introitus to 3 cm below the urethral meatus in continuity.

3. The bladder is reflected medially, leaving a full-thickness fibromuscular layer on the vaginal mucosa. The anterior dissection is continued laterally to ensure that the paravesical space is fully opened with full access under the ischiopubic ramus.

4. The pararectal space is opened with sharp dissection beginning at the introitus and mobilizing the rectum medially with the puborectalis muscle laterally and the sacrospinous ligament superiorly running from ischial spine to sacrum.

5. Anterior trocar incisions: The first incision is made at the genitofemoral fold at the level of the urethra; the second incision is made 3 cm lateral and below the ist incision.

6. Posterior trocar: Entry incisions are placed 3 cm lateral and inferior to the anus.

7. Insertion of anterior trocar: Beginning with the superior or deep trocar, the trocar is advanced straight until the pubic ramus is identified; the trocar is then rotated to pass behind the pubic ramus as close as possible to the ischial spine. In the paravaginal space, the Breisky-Navratil retractor guards the bladder, and the surgeon's second and third fingers are placed on the bladder surface of the pubic ramus; the trocar is then introduced between the surgeon's fingers to minimize any risk of the bladder mucosa being traversed. Once the tip of the trocar is safely introduced into paravesical space, the metal trocar is withdrawn and the blue retriever is introduced and clipped laterally away from the surgical site. The distal anterior trocar is introduced similarly, traversing the pubic ramus closer to the end of the pubic symphysis.

8. The posterior trocar is advanced parallel to the rectum through the ischiorectal fossa with the surgeon's other hand in the pararectal space and on the sacrospinous ligament. The progress of

the trocar is monitored as it transgluteally approaches the sacrospinous ligament and enters the pararectal space 2 cm medial to the ischial spine between the surgeon's second and third fingers. The rectum is guarded by the Breisky-Navratil retractor to minimize any risk of the rectal mucosa being inadvertently breached. Once the six cannulas and retrieval devises are in place, the mesh is introduced.

9. The surgeon's gloves are changed, and mesh handling is minimized to decrease any potential for contamination. Any bleeding is controlled with bipolar diathermy and the mesh is introduced by retrieving the six arms with the blue retrieval devices. Three arms on one side are retrieved first with the anterior distal arm next, followed by the deep anterior and the posterior arms. The process is repeated on the other side.

10. Once the mesh is introduced, excess mesh is trimmed. Frequently, 3 to 4 cm are trimmed from the posterior leaf. The mesh is tacked anteriorly to the paraurethral tissue and posteriorly to the distal rectovaginal fascia with 2.0 Vicryl sutures to ensure the anterior and posterior leafs of the mesh do not retract in the early postoperative period until the mesh is fixed in position.

11. Vaginal mucosa is closed with a 2.0 continuous Vicryl suture.

12. A rectal examination is performed to ensure the rectal mucosa is intact; a cystoscopic examination ensures that the ureters are patent and the bladder is intact.

13. Antibiotics are initiated, thromboembolic stockings are worn for 7 days, and self-administered enoxaparin sodium (Clexane) (20 mg) is injected daily for 5 days for every patient. Patients at high risk of thromboembolic events must complete an extended course of self-administered Clexane (40 mg).

14. The vaginal pack is removed at 6:00 AM after surgery, and the indwelling catheter is removed at 12:00 PM after surgery; a trial of void is started. In women with large vault eversions, the authors of this text leave the vaginal pack in for 48 hours to allow the vagina to be more fixed to the mesh initially; however, no evidence exists that supports this approach.

See Video 7-7, "Total Vaginal Mesh Procedure," for a video demonstration of a total mesh repair.

Case Discussion

Recognizing the superior outcomes of an LSC, as compared with the TVM technique, the authors of this text routinely perform an LSC in this type of patient. However, in patients not suitable for the laparoscopic approach, including those with significant medical co-morbidities, obesity, and multiple prior abdominal procedures, the TVM procedure remains an option.

Most of the discussion relating to POP and bladder function relates to stress urinary incontinence and bladder overactivity. This case highlights the problem of voiding dysfunction and POP. The incidence of preoperative-documented voiding difficulties in women undergoing apical compartment prolapse surgery is not insignificant and varies between 16% and 24%. (Maher et al, 2004; Elser et al, 2010) Limited data are available on the impact of prolapse surgery in women with preoperative voiding dysfunction; however, patients believe that correcting the prolapse will alleviate voiding dysfunction; fortunately, the authors of this text have found this belief to be true in 11 out of 14 (78%) patients; a *de novo* postoperative voiding dysfunction has also been observed in 5% of patients. Logically, lower flow rates and lower detrusor pressures would be indicators of an increased risk of persisting postoperative voiding dysfunction in those with a high postvoid residual preoperatively. Recently, Araki and associates (2009) suggested that the detrusor voiding pressure and flow rate were more relevant than the postvoid residual in determining ongoing voiding dysfunction postoperatively. Therefore in the patient with low detrusor pressure, low flow rate, and high residual urine on preoperative urodynamic testing and with preoperative urinary tract infections, the postoperative pathologic outcome is a poor contractility bladder with ineffective emptying. This patient is different from the woman with prolapse who has a raised residual urine preoperatively but is able to void to completion when the partially obstructed prolapse is reduced. The poor contractility bladder may arise in women who chronically strain to empty the bladder against a large prolapse similar to that observed in some men with large prostates. As of this writing, the woman illustrated in this case is 4 months postprocedure and is resigned to an ongoing CISC that was fully documented and discussed with her preoperatively. Preoperatively identifying women who may be at increased risk of ongoing and prolonged voiding dysfunction will help in counseling them to have realistic expectations regarding bladder function postoperatively and will also serve to protect the surgeon against claims that the surgery was the cause of the prolonged voiding dysfunction. The authors of this text perform full urodynamic analysis preoperatively in women with large prolapse in attempt to identify and document preoperative voiding dysfunction, bladder overactivity, and occult stress urinary incontinence with or without intrinsic sphincter deficiency. Preoperative risk factors for prolonged ongoing voiding difficulties postoperatively include large prolapse (extending 5 cm beyond the introitus), history of having to reduce prolapse to void or poor stream, history of recurrent urinary tract infections, high postvoid residual levels (more than 100 ml), and low flow rate and low detrusor pressure with voiding.

Case 4: Vaginal Hysterectomy, Uterosacral Colpopexy and Native Tissue Repair for Uterine Procidentia

A 67-year-old woman (para 3) has advanced uterovaginal prolapse and a significant cystocele, rectocele, and enterocele. Her cervix descends approximately 10 cm outside the introitus. She wants to maintain sexual activity. After detailed discussion of a variety of options, she decides to proceed with a vaginal hysterectomy, uterosacral colpopexy, and suture repair of the cystocele and rectocele without using any synthetic mesh **as shown in Video 7.8, "High Uterosacral Vaginal Vault Suspension Performed after Vaginal Hysterectomy."** Risks and benefits of this surgical procedure versus other potential techniques including ASC are discussed in great detail and appropriate consent forms are signed.

Procedural Details

1. This patient undergoes a vaginal hysterectomy; a large enterocele sac is addressed by excising the posterior vaginal wall, and the peritoneum is excised to reduce the caliber of the upper part of the posterior vaginal wall. If the patient had a posthysterectomy vault prolapse, the authors of this text believe it would have been mandatory to enter the peritoneum. Although extraperitoneal uterosacral suspension procedures have been described, in the authors' opinion, the appropriate structures are not easily identifiable unless performed via an intraperitoneal approach. Entering the peritoneum is obviously not an issue if the patient is undergoing a vaginal hysterectomy. If the patient has posthysterectomy prolapse, then the surgeon must be able to isolate an enterocele and enter the peritoneum. Once in the peritoneum, the cul-de-sac should be relatively free of any adhesive disease.

2. Packing the bowel: The next step is to pack the small bowel out of the cul-de-sac to allow easy access and visualization of the uppermost portions of the uterosacral ligament; this is best accomplished by passing large moistened laparotomy sponges intraperitoneally and then elevating these sponges with a large retractor such as a Deaver, Breisky-Navratil, or Sweetheartretractor. When the bowel is appropriately packed, the retractor will lift the intestinal contents out of the pelvis, usually allowing easy access to the proximal uterosacral ligaments.

3. Bilateral palpation of the ischial spines: Palpating the ischial spines is important. Many times the ureter can be palpated against the side wall as well. If the surgeon palpates the ischial spines and then continues to palpate in a medial and cephalad direction many times, then the C-SSL muscle complex can be palpated transperitoneally. If sutures can be passed at this level, then the result is usually a vagina that is approximately 9 cm in length.

4. Passage of sutures: Passage of the sutures through the uterosacral ligament complex is best performed by using a long needle holder and a Breisky-Navratil retractor. The Breisky-Navratil retractor is used to retract the sigmoid colon in the opposite direction. A light attached to a suction or retractor is also helpful. Elevating and applying traction on the distal uterosacral ligament allows visualization of the appropriate site for suture placement. The area of suture passage is identified by palpation, and the preference is to pass at least two sutures on each side. These sutures are then individually tagged. Delayed absorbable sutures are used because

bringing all of the sutures through the full thickness of the posterior vaginal wall is preferred. (The sutures are tied in the lumen of the vagina; thus a permanent suture would not be acceptable). Other modifications pass the sutures through the muscular layer of the vagina; in these situations, permanent sutures can be used. Once the sutures are brought through the full thickness of the posterior vaginal wall (including the peritoneum, if possible), they are then again individually tagged. If the anterior segment is well supported, then the vaginal incision is closed with a continuous delayed absorbable suture. The sutures are tied, elevating the apex into the hollow of the sacrum. If an anterior colporrhaphy is needed, as in this case, then the repair is performed and the anterior vaginal wall, as well as the vaginal cuff, is closed before tying the suspension sutures.

5. After tying the sutures, 5 ml intravenous (IV) indigo carmine is administered. In a patient with no renal compromise, the indigo carmine should be observed in the bladder in 5 to 10 minutes. If the patient is older or the surgeon wants to expedite this step, then 5 to 10 mg frusemide can be administered IV push. A cystoscopic examination is then performed to ensure ureteral patency. A spill of dye-colored urine from both ureteral orifices should be observed. If the dye does not spill after a reasonable time (usually 20 minutes), it can be assumed that the ureter on that side has been obstructed.

6. Complete vaginal reconstruction: The remainder of the procedures required to complete the surgery usually involves a posterior colporrhaphy and perineoplasty. The authors of this text also reserve any synthetic suburethral sling to be performed, if needed, after the vault procedure is completed.

See Figure 7-12 for an illustrative description of the various steps previously described for performing a high vaginal uterosacral vault suspension. (**See Video 7-9, "High Uterosacral Vaginal Vault Suspension for Posthysterectomy Prolapse,"** for a video demonstration of this procedure.)

Case Discussion

The concept of using the uterosacral ligaments for support of the vaginal cuff is not new. As early as 1957, Milton McCall (1957) described the McCall culdoplasty during which sutures incorporated the uterosacral ligaments into the posterior vaginal vault to obliterate the cul-de-sac and suspend and support the vaginal apex at the time of vaginal hysterectomy (see Chapter 4). In the early 1990s the late Cullen Richardson promoted the concept that, in patients with POP, the uterosacral ligaments do not become attenuated but rather break at specific points. Bob Shull et al (2000) took this idea and described how the procedure can be performed vaginally by passing sutures bilaterally through the uterosacral ligaments near the level of the ischial spine. Furthermore, modifications of the procedure have allowed a higher (more cephalad) and medial placement of sutures transperitoneally into the C-SSL complex. See Figures 7-13 and 7-14 for intraperitoneal and cross-sectional views of the placement of these various sutures. (**See Video 7-10, "High Intraperitoneal Vaginal Vault Suspension—Revisiting this Pelvic Anatomy"** for more detailed anatomic descriptions and examples of this procedure.) Since Shull's description, numerous publications have demonstrated outcomes similar to other vaginal suspension procedures such as sacrospinous ligament suspension. The potential advantages to the procedure are that it provides good apical support without significant distortion of the vaginal axis, making the procedure amendable to all types of vaginal prolapse. In addition, the intraperitoneal passage of sutures can be a lot cleaner and simpler than passing the sutures through the retroperitoneal structures such as the sacrospinous ligament. A disadvantage of the procedure is that the uterosacral ligament can, at times, come in close proximity to the ureter; studies have shown that the ureter can be easily kinked when these sutures are passed too far laterally.

This case demonstrates how a large primary prolapse can still be treated with a native tissue repair using sutures. Such a repair provides acceptable long-term durability with good quality-of-life improvements and minimal morbidity. (Baggish, Karram, 2011, Silva et al, 2006) Important technical aspects of the procedure include appropriate passage with sutures through the uppermost portion of the uterosacral ligament and the avoidance of any ureteral kinking that occurs in 2% to 5% of patients. When the ureter is kinked, intraoperative identification is mandatory; simply cutting the offending suture and then confirming the spill of indigo carmine is all that is required. The decision to replace the suture is made on an individual basis.

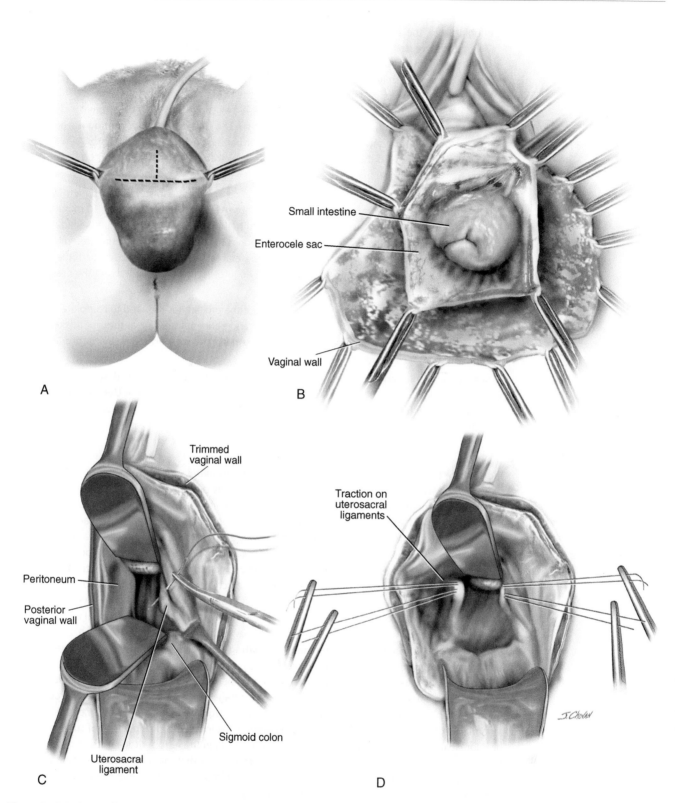

Figure 7-12 Technique for high uterosacral vaginal vault suspension (HUSLS). **A,** The most prominent portion of the prolapsed vaginal vault is grasped with two Allis clamps. **B,** The vaginal wall is opened up, and the enterocele sac is identified and entered. **C,** The bowel is packed high into the pelvis using large laparotomy sponges. The retractor lifts the sponges up out of the lower pelvis, thus completely exposing the cul-de-sac. When appropriate traction is placed downward on the uterosacral ligaments with an Allis clamp, the uterosacral ligaments are easily palpated bilaterally. **D,** Delayed absorbable sutures have been passed through the uppermost portion of the uterosacral ligaments on each side and have been individually tagged.

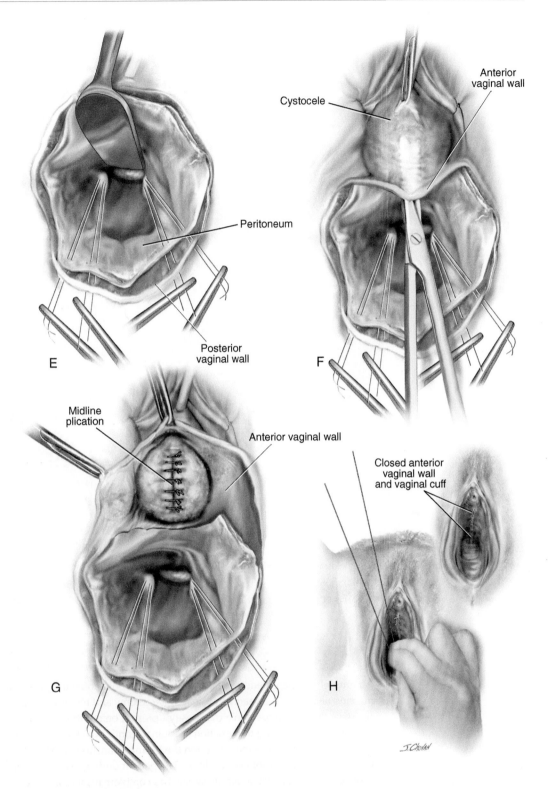

Figure 7-12, cont'd. E, Each end of the previously passed sutures is brought out through the posterior peritoneum and posterior vaginal wall. (A free needle is used to pass both ends of these delayed absorbable sutures through the full thickness of the vaginal wall.) **F,** The anterior colporrhaphy is begun by initiating a dissection between the prolapsed bladder and the anterior vaginal wall. **G,** Anterior colporrhaphy has been completed. **H,** The vagina has been appropriately trimmed and closed with interrupted or continuous delayed absorbable sutures. After the closure of the vagina, the delayed absorbable sutures that were previously brought out through the full thickness of the posterior vaginal wall are tied, thereby elevating the prolapsed vaginal vault high into the hollow of the sacrum.

(From Baggish MS, Karram MM: Atlas of pelvic anatomy and gynecologic surgery, *ed 3, St Louis, 2011, Elsevier.)*

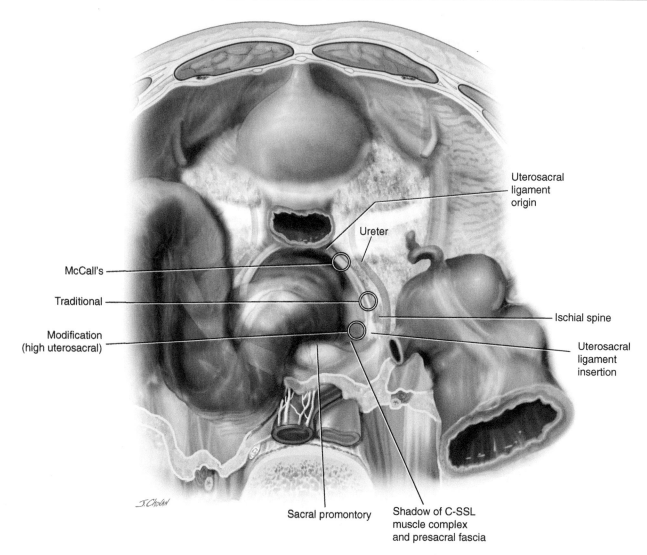

Figure 7-13 Intraperitoneal view of the uterosacral ligament with circles demonstrates suture placement for the McCall culdoplasty, traditional uterosacral suspension, and modified high uterosacral suspension. The close proximity of the ureter to the uterosacral ligament is noted.

(From Baggish MS, Karram MM: Atlas of pelvic anatomy and gynecologic surgery, *ed 3, St Louis, 2011, Elsevier.)*

Case 5: Vault Prolapse and Deep Dyspareunia

Patients with prolapse and significant dyspareunia pose some unique challenges in their surgical management. Within 2 years of vaginal hysterectomy and repair, a 58-year-old woman exhibits very significantly deep dyspareunia that was not present before the vaginal surgeries. An examination reveals no focal scarring or reduction in vaginal length, which might account for the deep dyspareunia. The vault is tender during the examination, and ultrasound imaging excludes any identifiable pelvic pathologic condition. The patient undergoes laparoscopic mobilization of the vaginal cuff and LSC. Postoperatively, she has complete resolution of her deep dyspareunia. (**See Video 7-11, "Laparoscopic Release of Vaginal Scarring Prior to Laparoscopic Colpopexy."**

Case Discussion

Recently, it is has been suggested that patients with dyspareunia before surgery are very likely to have dyspareunia after vaginal prolapse surgery, regardless of whether mesh is introduced. (Fatton, Lagrange, Jacquetin, 2010) This case highlights the benefits of the LSC in the management of patients with vault prolapse and deep dyspareunia. The procedure necessitates a full mobilization of the vaginal vault, which may be beneficial in this group of women.

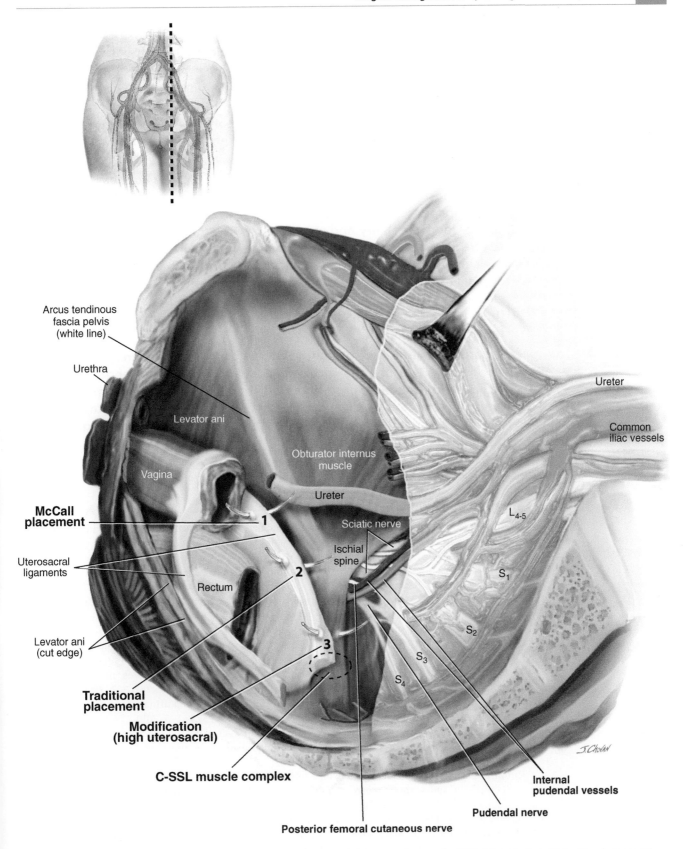

Arcus tendinous
fascia pelvis
(white line)

Urethra

Levator ani

Vagina

Obturator internus
muscle

Ureter

**McCall
placement** — 1

Sciatic nerve

Uterosacral
ligaments

Ischial
spine

Rectum

2

Levator ani
(cut edge)

3

**Traditional
placement**

**Modification
(high uterosacral)**

C-SSL muscle complex

Ureter

Common
iliac vessels

L4-5

S1

S2

S3

S4

Internal
pudendal vessels

Pudendal nerve

Posterior femoral cutaneous nerve

J. Chovan

Figure 7-14 Cross-section of the pelvic floor demonstrates the intraperitoneal placement of sutures for (1) McCall culdoplasty, (2) traditional uterosacral suspension, and (3) modified high uterosacral suspension. The high uterosacral suspension may involve the passage of the suture through the coccygeus–sacrospinous ligament (C-SSL) muscle complex, as a portion of the uterosacral ligament inserts into this structure.

(From Baggish MS, Karram MM: Atlas of pelvic anatomy and gynecologic surgery, ed 3, St Louis, 2011, Elsevier.)

SUMMARY: A competent reconstructive pelvic floor surgeon has a variety of surgical options available to manage apical compartment prolapse. The highlights of this chapter include the following:

- The sacral colpopexy is the current gold standard procedure for post hysterectomy vaginal vault prolapse; the authors of this text always perform this procedure laparoscopically. However, the surgeon requires a variety of options including vaginal approaches as outlined in this chapter for those patients not suitable for abdominal surgery.

- Currently, the ideal vaginal procedure for vault prolapse is not clear; many clinicians have strong views and prefer the vaginal approach. Both the sacrospinous colpopexy and uterosacral colpopexy have significant data detailing their success rates, durability, and complications. The transvaginal meshes are likely to provide satisfactory anatomic outcomes; however, less is known regarding their long-term outcomes and complications. Until more data are available, the authors of this text, if required to perform vaginal vault surgery, will initially elect native tissue vault suspensions and perhaps use transvaginal meshes for those with recurrent prolapse after failed native repairs and significant consultation with the patient.

- Regarding uterine prolapse, an extensive array of procedures is performed worldwide. Currently, the ideal management is unknown and can include vaginal and abdominal procedures with and without hysterectomy. With the rate of hysterectomy on the decline as a result of menorrhagia, the clinician will more frequently be asked to treat uterine prolapse; this area requires significantly more research.

Suggested Readings

Araki I, Haneda Y, Mikami Y, et al: Incontinence and detrusor dysfunction associated with pelvic organ prolapse: clinical value of preoperative urodynamic evaluation, *Int Urogynecol J Pelvic Floor Dysfunct* 20(11):1301–1306, 2009.

Baggish MS, Karram MM: Atlas of pelvic anatomy and gynecologic surgery, ed 3, St Louis, 2011, Elsevier.

Benson JT, Lucente V, McClellan E: Vaginal versus abdominal reconstructive surgery for the treatment of pelvic support defects: a prospective randomized study with long-term outcome evaluation, *Am J Obstet Gynecol* 175(6):1418–1421, 1996.

Caquant F, Collinet P, Debodinance P, et al: Safety of trans vaginal mesh procedure: retrospective study of 684 patients, *J Obstet Gynaecol Res* 34(4):449–456, 2008.

Diwadkar GB, Barber MD, Feiner B, et al: Complication and reoperation rates after apical vaginal prolapse surgical repair: a systematic review, *Obstet Gynecol* 113(2 Pt 1):367–373, 2009.

Elser DM, Moen MD, Stanford EJ, et al: Abdominal sacrocolpopexy and urinary incontinence: surgical planning based on urodynamics, *Am J Obstet Gynecol* 202(4):375.e1–5, 2010.

Fatton B, Amblard J, Debodinance P, et al: Transvaginal repair of genital prolapse: preliminary results of a new tension-free vaginal mesh (Prolift technique)—a case series multicentric study, *Int Urogynecol J Pelvic Floor Dysfunct* 18(7):743–752, 2007.

Fatton B, Lagrange E, Jacquetin B: Sexual outcome after transvaginal repair of pelvic organ prolapse (POP) with and without mesh: A prospective study of 323 patients, Available at http://www.icsoffice.org/Abstracts/Publish/105/000053.pdf. Accessed 2010.

Haylen BT, de Ridder D, Freeman RM, et al: An International Urogynecological Association (IUGA)/International Continence Society (ICS) joint report on the terminology for female pelvic floor dysfunction, *Int Urogynecol J* 21(1):5–26, 2010.

Higgs PJ, Chua HL, Smith AR: Long term review of laparoscopic sacrocolpopexy, *BJOG* 112(8):1134–1138, 2005.

Iglesia CB,. Sokol AI, Sokol ER, et al: Vaginal mesh for prolapse: a randomized controlled trial, *Obstet Gynecol* 116(2 Pt 1):293–303, 2010.

Jundt K, Wagner S, von Bodungen V, et al: Occult incontinence in women with pelvic organ prolapse—Does it matter? *Eur J Med Res* 15(3):112–116, 2010.

Klauschie JL, Suozzi BA, O'Brien MM, et al: A comparison of laparoscopic and abdominal sacral col-popexy: objective outcome and perioperative differences, *Int Urogynecol J Pelvic Floor Dysfunct* 20(3):273–279, 2009.

Lo TS, Wang AC: Abdominal colposacropexy and sacrospinous ligament suspension for severe utero-vaginal prolapse: a comparison, *J Gynecol Surg* 14:59–64, 1998.

Maher C, Baessler K, Glazener CM, et al: Surgical management of pelvic organ prolapse in women, *Cochrane Database Syst Rev* 4:CD004014, 2007.

Maher C, Feiner B, Baessler K, et al: Surgical management of pelvic organ prolapse in women, *Cochrane Database Syst Rev* 4:CD004014, 2010.

Maher CF, Qatawneh AM, Dwyer PL, et al: Abdominal sacral colpopexy or vaginal sacrospinous col-popexy for vaginal vault prolapse: a prospective randomized study, *Am J Obstet Gynecol* 190(1):20–26, 2004.

Maher CF, Feiner B, DeCuyper EM, et al: Laparoscopic sacral colpopexy versus total vaginal mesh for the management of vaginal vault prolapse: a randomised controlled trial, *Am J Obstet Gynecol* 204(4):360.e1–e7, 2011.

Margulies RU, Rogers MA, Morgan DM: Outcomes of transvaginal uterosacral ligament suspension: systematic review and metaanalysis, *Am J Obstet Gynecol* 202(2):124–134, 2010.

McCall ML: Posterior culdeplasty; surgical correction of enterocele during vaginal hysterectomy; A preliminary report, *Obstet Gynecol* 10(6):595–602, 1957.

Milani AL, Withagen MI, Vierhout ME: Trocar-guided total tension-free vaginal mesh repair of post-hysterectomy vaginal vault prolapse, *Int Urogynecol J Pelvic Floor Dysfunct* 20(10):1203–1211, 2009.

North CE, Ali-Ross NS, Smith AR, et al: A prospective study of laparoscopic sacrocolpopexy for the management of pelvic organ prolapse, *BJOG* 116(9):1251–1257, 2009.

Nygaard IE, McCreery R, Brubaker L, et al: Abdominal sacrocolpopexy: a comprehensive review, *Obstet Gynecol* 104(4):805–823, 2004.

Paraiso MF, Walters MD, Rackley RR, et al: Laparoscopic and abdominal sacral colpopexies: a compara-tive cohort study, *Am J Obstet Gynecol* 192(5):1752–1758, 2005.

Paraiso MF, Jelovsek JE, Frick A, et al: Laparoscopic compared with robotic sacrocolpopexy for vaginal prolapse: a randomized controlled trial, *Obstet Gynecol* 118(5):1005–1013, 2011.

Rondini C, Alvarez M, Urzua R, Villegas M: Prospective randomised study comparing high uterosacral colpopexy for the correction of apical defects, *Int Urogynecol J* 22(Suppl I):S87–S88, 2011.

Sanses TV, Shahryarinejad A, Molden S, et al: Anatomic outcomes of vaginal mesh procedure (Prolift) compared with uterosacral ligament suspension and abdominal sacrocolpopexy for pelvic organ prolapse: a Fellows' Pelvic Research Network study, *Am J Obstet Gynecol* 201(5):519.e511–518, 2009.

Shull BL, Bachofen C, Coates KW, et al: A transvaginal approach to repair of apical and other associ-ated sites of pelvic organ prolapse with uterosacral ligaments, *Am J Obstet Gynecol* 2000;183:1365–1374, 2000.

Silva WA, Pauls RN, Segal JL, et al: Uterosacral ligament vault suspension: five-year outcomes, *Obstet Gynecol* 108:255–263, 2006.

Withagen MI, Milani AL, den Boon J, et al: Trocar-guided mesh compared with conventional vaginal repair in recurrent prolapse: A randomized controlled trial, *Obstet Gynecol* 117(2 Pt 1):242–250, 2011.

Surgical Management of Anterior Vaginal Wall Prolapse

Christopher F. Maher MD and Mickey Karram MD

 Video Clips online

Introduction

In 1909, White stated that the only unresolved problem in plastic gynecology was the permanent cure of cystocele (White, 1909). Today, the surgical management of anterior compartment prolapse remains problematic and controversial. Anterior compartment prolapse is the most common site of prolapse and the site of prolapse with the highest anatomic failure rate with a plethora of surgical options available to the clinician. The goal of this chapter is to provide an overview of the current literature and to discuss and demonstrate numerous approaches to the surgical management of anterior compartment prolapse.

Anterior vaginal wall prolapse, commonly termed *cystocele*, is defined as the pathologic descent of the anterior vaginal wall overlying the bladder base. Cystocele may frequently co-exist with a variety of micturition disorders. The most contemporary understanding of the anatomy and support of this segment of the pelvic floor stems from concepts proposed by Richardson 1976, who described transverse, midline, and paravaginal defects. Transverse defects were said to occur when the pubocervical fascia separated from its insertion around the cervix; midline defects represented an antero-posterior separation of the fascia between the bladder and the vagina; and paravaginal defects represented a detachment of the lateral connective tissue attachments at the arcus tendineus fascia pelvis (ATFP). A conceptual representation of these various defects viewed from the retropubic space is shown in Figure 8-1.

All types of micturition disorders can be observed with anterior vaginal wall prolapse, and, to date, no clear scientific explanation exists to help clinicians understand the correlation between the anatomic descent of the anterior vaginal wall and the

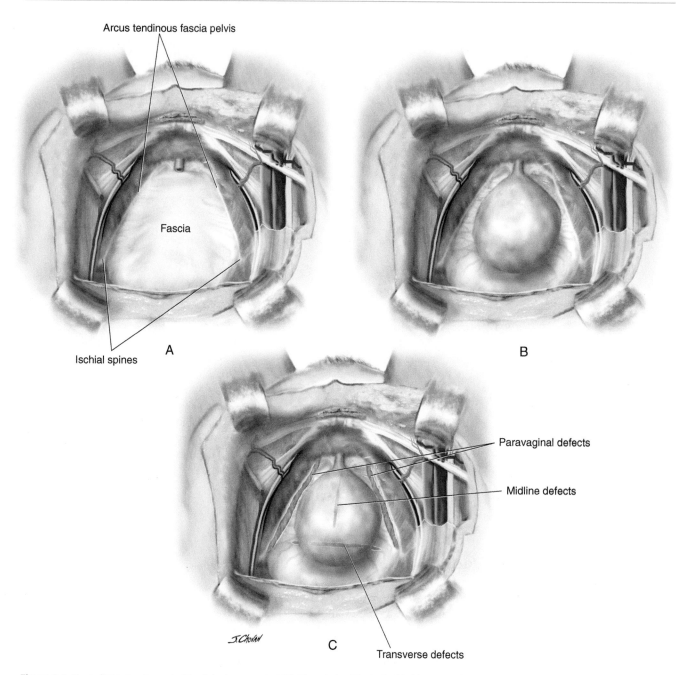

Figure 8-1 Normal intact pubocervical fascia is demonstrated **(A)**. The relationship to the bladder is visualized **(B)** and represents paravaginal, midline, and transverse defects **(C)**.

functional derangements of the urinary tract. When evaluating and planning the surgical management of patients with anterior vaginal wall descent, determining how the surgical intervention will affect any potential functional derangements that the patient may be experiencing is important. This aspect of the preoperative discussion with the patient and the consent process is extremely important. Although many surgeons have gone to great lengths to predict preoperatively what types of defect exist in patients with symptomatic anterior wall descent, the literature suggests that doing so is difficult to do, and, in reality, the determination of the various defects in the authors' opinion is an intraoperative finding with questionable clinical utility. Although numerous types of repairs are discussed and demonstrated in great detail in this chapter, the ultimate goal of any anterior vaginal wall support procedure is to recreate a trapezoid of support that mimics the pubocervical fascia and stems from below the proximal urethra to the

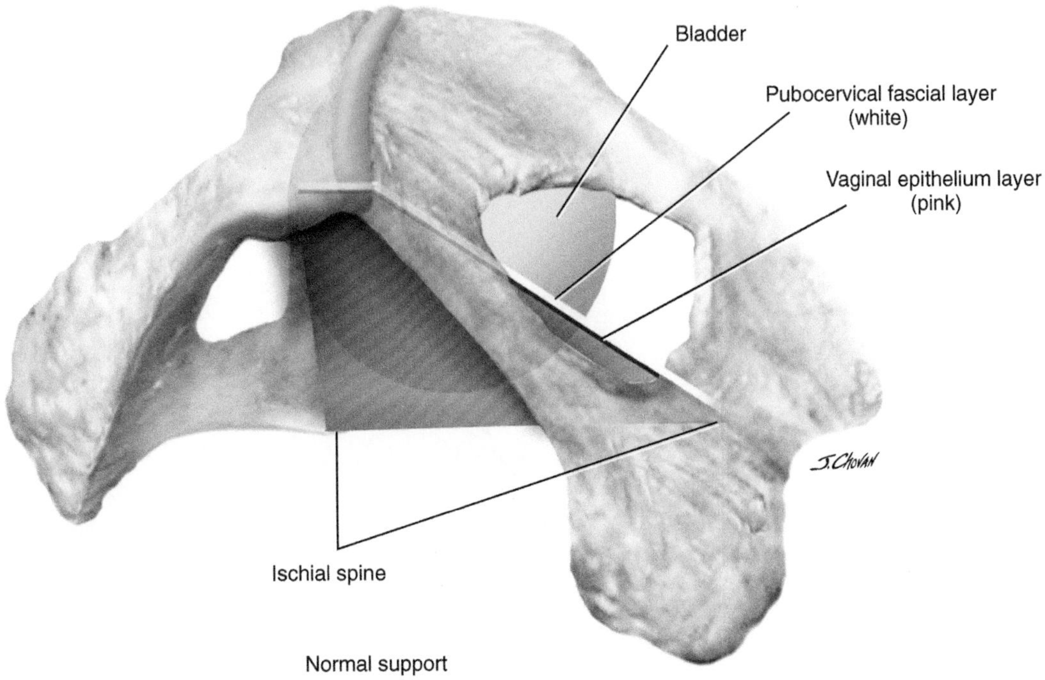

Figure 8-2 Normal anterior vaginal wall support is illustrated.

cervix or apex and laterally to the ATFP or fascia of the obturator internus muscle (Figure 8-2).

Finally, the long-term success of anterior vaginal wall repair is directly correlated with the ability to suspend the apex in a high, durable position without creating any significant distortion of the vaginal axis.

Background

In 1913, Kelly described the plication of the urethral sphincter muscle and the anterior colporrhaphy was born. The success rates of anterior colporrhaphy in the management of cystocele range from 80% to 100% in retrospective series. (Macer, 1978; Stanton et al, 1982; Walter et al, 1982; Porges, Smilen, 1994) More recently, Weber and colleagues (2001) and Sand and associates (2001) in randomized controlled trials (RCTs) reported anterior colporrhaphy to be successful in the management of cystocele in only 42% and 57% of cases, respectively.

White (1912) demonstrated the importance of paravaginal defects in anterior compartment prolapse. Richardson, Lyon, Williams (1976) described a series of defects in the pubocervical fascia, explaining why no single repair should be indiscriminately applied to all anterior compartment defects. He also advocated the abdominal paravaginal repair (Figure 8-3), which has a reported success rate of 75% to 97% in numerous case series. (Richardson, Lyon, Williams, 1976; Richardson, Edmonds, Williams, 1981; Shull, Baden, 1989; Scotti et al, 1998; Bruce, El Galley, Galloway, 1999) The surgical technique of the laparoscopic paravaginal repair is well described, but little information is available on the efficacy of this approach.

Shull and colleagues (1994) also reported on the safety and efficacy of the transvaginal paravaginal repair (Figure 8-4) in 1994. Although the success rates of the transvaginal paravaginal repair for cystocele in case series vary from 67% to 100% (White, 1912; Shull, Benn, Kuehl, 1994; Grody et al, 1995; Elkins et al, 2000; Mallipeddi et al, 2001; Young, Daman, Bony, 2001), significant complications have been reported. Mallipeddi reported on complications in a series of 45 patients including one bilateral ureteric obstruction, one retropubic hematoma requiring surgery, two vaginal abscesses, and

Figure 8-3 Abdominal paravaginal repair reattaches the fascia to the white line.

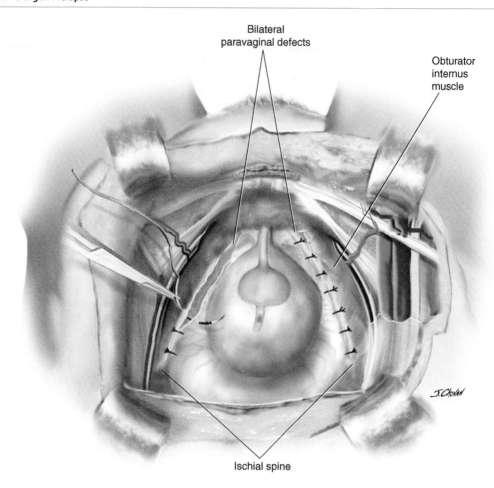

Bilateral paravaginal defects

Obturator internus muscle

Ischial spine

two transfusions. In a series of 100 women, Young, Daman, Bony (2001) reported 21 major complications and a 16% transfusion rate.

In line with our surgical colleagues who moved to utilise mesh in hernia repairs, in the last decade there has been to move toward graft prosthesis in prolapse surgery. This movement took much of its impetus from two early papers. Olsen 1997 reported a reoperation rate of 29% after prolapse and/or continence surgery; Weber reported a 70% failure rate of native tissue in anterior compartment repair. A recent re-evaluation of Olsen's same demographic criteria 10 years later revealed a more acceptable re-operation rate of 17% (Denman et al, 2008). In addition, a recent re-analysis of Weber's data using a less strict definition of objective success reveals outcomes to be considerably better than originally reported with only 10% of patients developing anatomic recurrence beyond the hymen, 5% developing symptomatic recurrence, and reoperation rates less than 1% at 23-months' follow-up. (Chmielewski et al, 2011) These re-evaluations 10 years after the primary publications challenge the reasoning that validates the introduction of transvaginal polypropylene mesh augmentation.

Historically, clinicians have sought more durable repairs. Julian and colleagues (1996) demonstrated in a prospective case control study that women who underwent at least two previous vaginal repairs, the overlaying of a Marlex (Bard) mesh to the anterior colporrhaphy reduced the recurrence rate of cystocele from 33% to 0%. The Marlex mesh was associated with a mesh erosion rate of 25%. In a retrospective review of 142 women with Marlex mesh augmentation of the anterior colporrhaphy, Flood, Drutz, Waja (1998) demonstrated a 100% success rate for cystoceles at a 3.2-year follow-up and a mesh erosion rate of only 2%. Although the Marlex mesh has largely been abandoned, the great variation in reported outcomes (e.g., mesh exposures in these two papers), highlighted the ongoing problem with polypropylene meshes 15 years earlier.

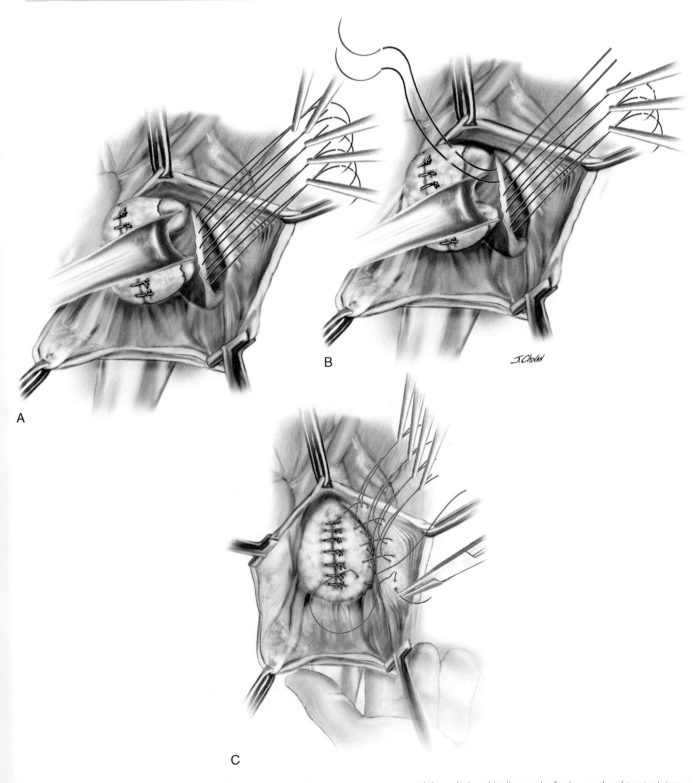

A

B

J. Chovan

C

Figure 8-4 Surgical steps for vaginal paravaginal (3-point) repair. **A,** Numerous sutures are passed through the white line on the fascia over the obturator internus muscle (point 1). **B,** Each suture is passed through the lateral edge of the detached fascia (point 2). **C,** Each suture is passed through the full thickness of the vaginal wall excluding the epithelium (point 3).

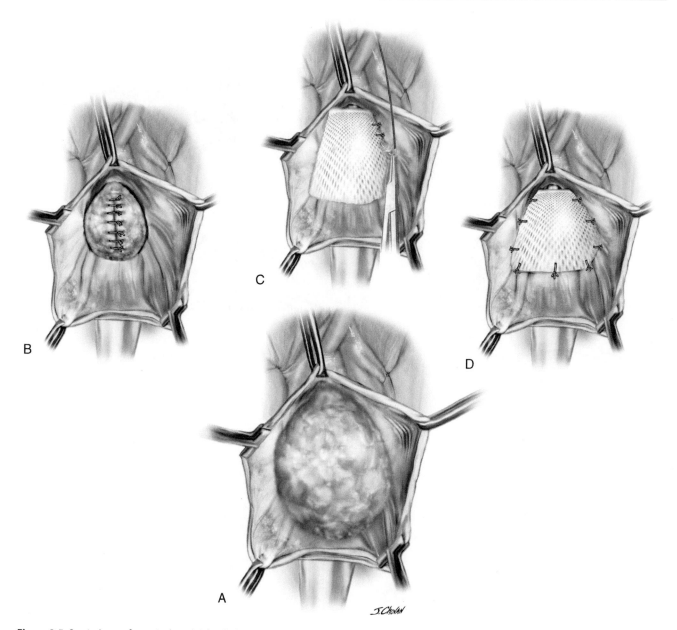

Figure 8-5 Surgical steps for vaginal mesh inlay. **A,** Anterior compartment prolapse is visualized. **B,** Midline fascial plication is demonstrated. **C-D,** Self-styled mesh is sutured in place. (**See Video 8-1, "Anterior Colporrhaphy with Biologic Mesh Augmentation,"** for a video demonstration.)

The 2012 Cochrane review concluded that polyglactin (Vicryl) absorbable mesh in the management of anterior compartment prolapse, as compared with anterior colporrhaphy alone, is more likely to be successful (relative risk [RR] 1.39, 95%; confidence interval [CI] 1.02 to 1.90). Only one case of mesh removal has been reported. A variety of permanent meshes has also been evaluated, and the data from three trials demonstrate that anterior vaginal repair using polypropylene mesh overlay (Figure 8-5) was superior in reducing anterior compartment recurrences on objective assessment, compared with native tissue anterior colporrhaphy (RR 2.14, 95%; CI 1.23 to 3.74).

Transobturator-armed polypropylene meshes, either self-styled or kits, had a lower rate of anterior compartment prolapse on examination, as compared with anterior colporrhaphy alone (RR 3.51, 95%; CI 2.71 to 4.02). After transvaginal polypropylene mesh augmentation, women also had a superior subjective success rate (RR 1.57, 95%; CI 1.18 to 2.07), as compared with anterior colporrhaphy. Further prolapse surgery was not significantly more common after anterior colporrhaphy—14 out of 459 patients (3%), as compared with 6 out of 470 patients (1.3%) after transobturator polypropylene mesh (RR 2.18, 95%; CI 0.93 to 5.10). No difference was detected in individual studies in validated prolapse-specific questions, and metaanalysis was not possible because of the variations in the questionnaires. The surgical time and blood loss were significantly greater in the mesh group, and a tendency toward lower cystotomy rates was reported (0.4% versus 2.7% [RR 0.19, 95%; CI 0.03 to 1.07]) (Altman et al, 2011; Nieminen et al, 2010), *de novo* dyspareunia (4% versus 8% [RR 0.51, 95%; CI 0.21 to 1.23]), and *de novo* stress urinary incontinence (SUI) (7.3% versus 11.4% [RR 0.65, 95%; CI 0.4 to 1.07]) after anterior colporrhaphy. (Altman et al, 2011, Sivaslioglu, Unlubilgin, Dolen, 2008; Nieminen et al, 2010) Continence surgery was performed in similar numbers in both groups, 15 of 368 women after anterior colporrhaphy and 12 of 380 women after polypropylene mesh procedure (RR 1.29, 95%; CI 0.63 to 2.63). Metaanalysis of those studies that reported *de novo* prolapse in the apical or posterior compartment found a lower rate after the anterior colporrhaphy (14 of 147 patients [9.5%]), as compared with transobturator mesh (26 of 148 patients [17.7%]) (RR 0.49, 95%; CI 0.24 to 0.97). Mesh erosions were reported in 41 of 393 women (10.4%) who had an anterior compartment polypropylene mesh, and surgical intervention occurred in 34 of 540 women (6.3%) to correct mesh erosion.

In the surgical management of anterior compartment prolapse, a plethora of surgical options are available. The following cases demonstrate the authors' surgical approach to common anterior compartment clinical scenarios, with the goal of providing justifications to the approach in the case discussions.

Case 1: Anterior Repair with Midline Fascial Plication

 View: Videos 8-2 and 8-3

A 55-year-old woman has moderate symptomatic anterior compartment prolapse that approaches the vaginal introitus with straining. She has no other associated urinary or bowel symptoms. Vaginal examination reveals that the anterior compartment extends to within 1 cm of the introitus with the uterus and posterior compartment remaining well supported. With a reduction of the anterior prolapse, no occult stress incontinence is identified. She has undergone no prior pelvic surgeries. The patient has consented to a midline plication of the cystocele (Figure 8-6) with a Kelly-Kennedy plication of the bladder neck (Figure 8-7).

Surgical Steps
The important steps of the procedure are presented as follows (see Figure 8-6):

1. Tenaculums are placed on the midline anterior vaginal wall just below the urethra and at the vaginocervical junction.

2. A midline incision is made in the vaginal mucosa.

3. The authors of this text prefer to use no local anesthetic or hydrodistention, thus allowing a clear demarcation of the planes.

4. Artery forceps are attached to the vaginal mucosa to aid in dissection. An assistant uses forceps to aid in traction to demonstrate the appropriate fascial plane. The surgeon holds Metzenbaum scissors in the dominant hand, and the nondominant hand is positioned under the vaginal mucosa to maximize traction and minimize the risk of "button-holing" the vagina during dissection.

5. With traction and countertraction in the appropriate plane, dissection starts; the fascial tissue is quickly mobilized from the vagina bilaterally. The bladder is also mobilized from the cervix to allow fixation of the fascial repair to the proximal anterior cervix, which, in this case, is well supported.

6. The dissection extends laterally to the inferior pubic ramus, and good paravaginal support is confirmed.

7. Central plication begins at the proximal urethra with a series of interrupted 0 polydioxanone sutures (PDSs). Some surgeons routinely place Kelly-Kennedy plication sutures at the level of

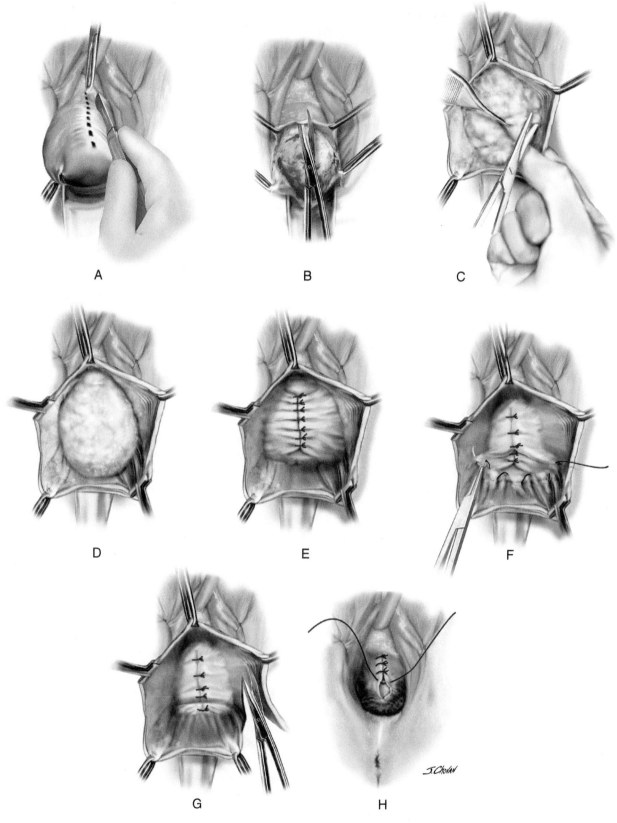

Figure 8-6 Classical anterior colporrhaphy. **A,** Initial midline anterior vaginal wall incision is demonstrated. **B,** The midline incision is extended using scissors. **C,** Sharp dissection of the bladder off the vaginal wall should be lateral to the superior pubic ramus, and the base of the bladder should be dissected off the vaginal cuff or cervix to the level of the preperitoneal space of the anterior cul-de-sac. **D,** The bladder has been completely mobilized off the vagina. **E,** Initial plication layer is placed. **F,** Second plication layer is placed, which commonly requires further mobilization of vaginal muscularis off of the vaginal epithelium. The most proximal stitch involves plication of the inside of the vaginal wall at the level of the vaginal apex or upper portion of the cervix. **G,** The completed second plication layer and the trimming of excess vaginal mucosa are demonstrated. **H,** Closure of vaginal mucosa is demonstrated.

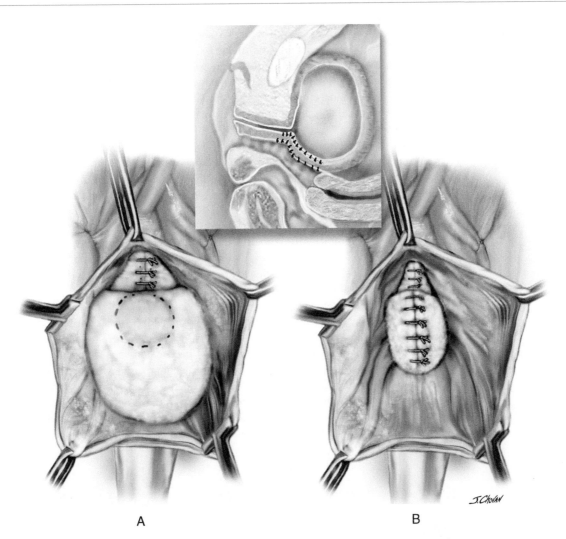

A   B

Figure 8-7 Anterior colporrhaphy with Kelly-Kennedy plication. **A,** Vaginal mucosa is opened, and interrupted sutures are started under the urethra. **B,** Completed colporrhaphy uses midline plication with interrupted sutures. Preferential support is provided to the proximal urethra over that provided to the bladder neck.

the proximal urethra and bladder neck in all patients with urethral hypermobility with no evidence of occult incontinence (see Figure 8-7). These sutures are designed to provide preferential support to the bladder neck over that of the bladder base. The final sutures incorporate the fascia and cervical tissue.

8. A continuous locking delayed absorbable suture closes the vaginal mucosa and includes a central bite in the plicated fascia layer.

9. Cystoscopic examination ensures that the bladder mucosa has not been breached and that the ureters are patent.

10. Vaginal packing and an indwelling catheter are placed. Packing is removed at 6:00 AM the following morning after surgery, and a voiding trial is performed before discharge.

(**See Video 8-2, "Anterior Repair with Midline Fascial Plication,"** and **Video 8-3, "Anterior Colporrhaphy with Kelly Plication,"** for demonstrations of anterior colporrhaphy with midline fascial plication and anterior colporrhaphy with Kelly-Kennedy plication.)

Case Discussion

The traditional well-performed anterior colporrhaphy is ideal in this scenario with an isolated anterior compartment prolapse (see Figures 8-6 and 8-7). The role of routinely performing a Kelly-Kennedy plication in such a setting is controversial and currently based on surgeon preference. The theoretical advantage is that the surgeon may be reducing the rate of *de novo* development of SUI; however, to date no studies have truly objectified this potential advantage. The incorporation of the fascial repair into the firm proximal anterior cervical tissue (Video 8-2) or durable tissue at the level of the vaginal cuff after hysterectomy serves to connect the level 2 fascial repair; the cervix or vaginal cuff serves as the central cornerstone of the fascial tissue in the upper vagina with the anterior and posterior compartment fascia and the uterosacral, cardinal, and broad ligaments all attaching (Figure 8-8).

The importance of the apical compartment in the causes of anterior compartment prolapse cannot be underestimated, and Delancey in 2006 demonstrated that up to 50% of anterior compartment prolapse is a result of apical prolapse. (Summers et al, 2006) On linear regression, modeling found that 77% of anterior wall descent can be explained by apical descent and midsagittal anterior vaginal wall length. (Hsu et al, 2008) In the 2008 International Collaboration on Incontinence on Surgical Management of Prolapse, an expert panel stated that "… apical compartment support remains the cornerstone of successful prolapse surgery," (Brubaker et al, 2005) and the authors would rarely perform an anterior compartment defect in isolation. Suffice it to say, a large prolapse in one compartment should not dictate the surgery performed in all compartments. **See Video 8-4, "Large Prolapse Suitable for Anterior Colporrhaphy,"** demonstrates that while a patient may have significant uterine and posterior compartment defects the anterior compartment remains relatively well supported and this patient is ideally placed for anterior colporrhaphy incorporated to the anterior lip of the distal cervix, sacrospinous hysteropexy and posterior colporrhaphy. The author of this text retains the use transvaginal polypropylene mesh for those patients with large or recurrent anterior compartment prolapse who have the uterus present. The higher risk of anatomic failure associated with the native tissue repair may offset the increased risk of blood loss and mesh complication rates associated with the polypropylene transobturator meshes. This approach should continue to be monitored as more data become available on long-term success rates and complications associated with vaginal grafts in the anterior compartment.

Case 2: Laparoscopic Paravaginal Repair

View: Video 8-5

A 45-year-old woman has moderate anterior compartment prolapse; the uterus and posterior compartment are well supported. No symptoms of bladder dysfunction are revealed, and she has undergone no previous surgeries. This patient was considered to be a good candidate for a paravaginal repair, which provides lateral anterior vaginal wall support (Figure 8-9).

In conjunction with this surgery in those patients with urinary stress incontinence, the medial two sutures are secured to the more robust pectineal ligament. The abdominal paravaginal repair is also ideal for correcting the urethroceles, which can be difficult to address vaginally because of the paucity of good paraurethral tissue. A paravaginal repair is commonly performed in conjunction with sacral colpopexy if anterior vaginal wall support is needed. The laparoscopic approach to paravaginal repair affords many benefits including excellent vision in the Retzius cavity, magnification, and positive intraabdominal pressure that aids in dissection and hemostasis; this approach is also ideal for teaching.

Surgical Steps

1. An open Hassan subumbilical entry is performed with the introduction of a 10-mm trocar. The authors of this text prefer a 0-degree scope; however, many clinicians use a 30-degree scope.

2. Two additional 5-mm secondary trocars are introduced: (a) skin incisions 2 cm medial and lateral to anterior superior iliac crest; and (b) entry into the peritoneal cavity under vision and lateral to the inferior epigastric vessels.

3. The Retzius cavity is entered with the peritoneum incised with monopolar diathermy just below the junction of the medial umbilical ligaments. The incisions continue laterally to the median umbilical ligament and then parallel to the median umbilical ligament toward the insertion of the round ligament to the pelvic side wall. This opening technique ensures that the surgeon

Figure 8-8 The cervix serves as the central cornerstone of the fascial tissue in the upper vagina with the anterior and posterior compartment fascia and the uterosacral, cardinal, and broad ligaments all attaching.

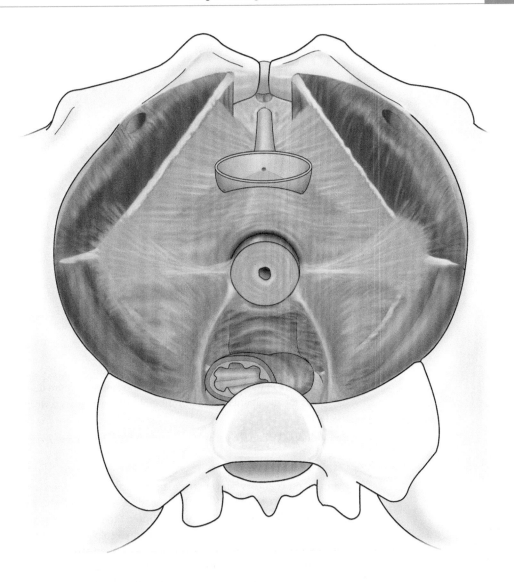

remains lateral to the bladder and medial to the inferior epigastric vessels. (**See Video 7-1, "Laparoscopic Trocar Placement Used for Reconstructive Surgical Procedures"** for a demonstration.)

4. The so-called champagne layer of the Retzius cavity is opened with gentle traction in primary cases or sharp dissection in those with previous surgery.

5. Using nontraumatic swabs and gentle traction, the paravesical spaces are bilaterally opened to display the ATFP running from the pubic symphysis medially toward the ischial spine laterally. The surgeon's left forefinger elevates the vagina after the bladder has been medially swept with the nontraumatic swabs in the surgeon's right hand to maximize exposure and safe access to the paravaginal tissue.

6. An Ethibond continuous suture (0.0) closes the arcus tendineus to the detached vaginal mucosa, starting laterally and working medially and then back again to tie the suture laterally. If the dissection is adequate, the bladder mucosa will not be breached. Full thickness bites of the vaginal mucosa should be avoided, which may result in granuloma or sinus formation in the vagina.

7. Cystoscopic examination is performed to ensure ureteral patency and to confirm that the bladder mucosa has not been traversed.

8. Vaginal packing, sequential compression devices, and indwelling catheter are removed the next day, and a trial of void is started.

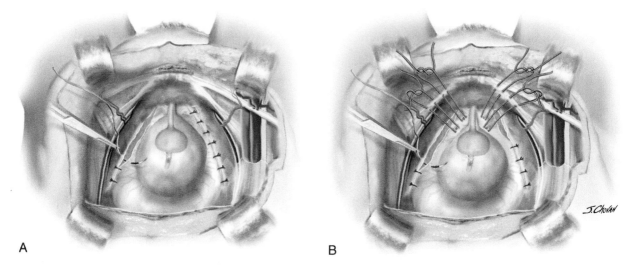

Figure 8-9 A, Paravaginal repair; the anterior pelvic fascia is being re-attached to the white line. **B,** In those patients with associated urinary stress incontinence, the medial two sutures are secured to pectineal ligament.

9. Antibiotics are initiated, self-administered enoxaparin sodium (Clexane) (20 mg) is injected daily for 5 days for all patients, and thromboembolic stockings are worn for 7 days as per preoperative risk factors.

See Video 8-5, "Laparoscopic Paravaginal Repair," for a video demonstration.

Case Discussion

This surgical procedure is rarely performed in isolation. In women with urinary stress incontinence and anterior compartment defects, the procedure is modified with a lateral suture that attaches the vagina to the ATFP, and medially two interrupted Ethibond sutures suspend the vagina to the pectineal ligament, as performed in the traditional colposuspension technique (see Figure 8-9, *B*).

More frequently, the paravaginal repair is performed after a sacral colpopexy as part of a total vaginal prolapse correction. Some clinicians now report sacral colpopexy performed with suburethral tapes for continence. Surgeons should be mindful that in the three RCTs that demonstrated the superiority of sacral colpopexy over vaginal surgery, anatomic support of the anterior compartment was sustained with either colposuspension or paravaginal repair at the time of sacral colpopexy in nearly 70% of the cases. Surgeons who choose to neglect the anterior compartment support afforded by paravaginal repair or colposuspension at the time of sacral colpopexy may risk exposing their patients to higher rates of failure.

Case 3: Uterovaginal Prolapse with Occult Stress Urinary Incontinence

  View: Video 8-6

A 67-year-old woman has significant uterovaginal prolapse extending 5 cm beyond the introitus that is uncomfortable and embarrassing to the patient. No associated bladder or bowel symptoms are revealed on examination; the prolapse is reduced digitally and occult stress urinary incontinence is identified. (**See Video 8-6, "Demonstration of Occult Incontinence,"** for a video demonstration of the technique used to reduce prolapse to test for occult stress incontinence). The patient is informed that the current use of synthetic mesh in the anterior compartment reduces the risk of recurrent anterior compartment prolapse, as compared with native tissue repair, by a factor of three with the principle risk factor being mesh erosion at a rate of 10%. (Maher et al, 2010)

Surgical Steps of Anterior Transobturator Mesh as Part of Hysteropexy

1. Hydrodissection with Marcaine solution 0.25% with adrenalin is introduced submucosally and in the paravesical space.

2. A midline vaginal incision is made from the cervix to 2 to 3 cm below the urethral meatus.

3. Artery forceps are placed on the vaginal mucosa to assist with traction. The surgeon holds Metzenbaum scissors in the dominant hand, and countertraction is achieved with Gillies forceps in the surgeon's nondominant hand. Dissection just below the vaginal mucosa and continuing to the pubic rami is identified, which is a wider dissection than performed for a traditional native tissue anterior colporrhaphy and may explain the increased blood loss reported with transobturator meshes, as compared with traditional anterior repair in the authors' recent Cochrane review. (Maher et al, 2010) Blunt finger dissection is used at the completion to ensure adequate is available to safely introduce the obturator trocars.

4. The bladder is also mobilized from the cervix to ensure that the mesh can be secured to the cervix at the completion of the surgery.

5. Two trocars incisions are made; the first incision is made in the genitofemoral fold at the level of the urethra, and the second for the deep arm is made 2 cm lateral and 2 cm below this point.

6. The trocars are introduced through the obturator space to the paravesical space with tactile sensation, and a Breisky-Navratil retractor reflects the bladder and minimizes any risk of perforating the bladder with the trocars. The trocars are designed to enter the paravesical space at the origin and in the section of the ATFP to offer a wide area of support to the central mesh.

7. Once the four trocars are safely established, the mesh is introduced beneath the bladder by retrieving the arms of the mesh through the trocars.

8. Initial tensioning of the mesh is performed with traction on the arms to bring the mesh in close proximity to the bladder.

9. A 2.0 Vicryl suture tacks the distal mesh to the vagina just lateral to the urethra with care to ensure that the vaginal mucosa has not been breached.

10. The tail of the mesh may be trimmed and sutured (2.0 Vicryl) to the anterior lip of the distal cervix from which the bladder has been previously mobilized (Figure 8-10).

11. The vaginal mucosa is closed with a continuous 2.0 Vicryl suture. A small amount of the vaginal mucosa is rarely trimmed if the prolapse is large.

12. Final tensioning of the mesh occurs after completing the surgery (i.e., hysteropexy and native tissue posterior repair). No excessive tension is placed on the mesh at the completion of the surgery. By placing digital pressure, which elevates the lateral vaginal mucosa above the pubic rami while the trocars or sleeve is removed on that side, no excessive tension is placed on the mesh body or arms.

13. Cystoscopic examination is performed to ensure ureteral patency and to confirm that the bladder mucosa has not been breached.

14. Vaginal packing, sequential compression devices, and the indwelling catheter are removed the next day, and a trial of void is started.

15. Antibiotics are initiated, self-administered enoxaparin sodium (Clexane) (20 mg) is injected daily for 5 days for all patients, and thromboembolic stockings are worn for 7 days as per preoperative risk factors.

See Video 8-7, "Anterior Prolift Sacrospinous Hysteropexy Posterior Repair," and Video 8-8, "Sacrospinous Hysteropexy, Anterior Perigee Mesh, Posterior Repair Tension-Free Vaginal Tape—the Transobturator Approach," 🎥 for video demonstrations of both the anterior Prolift and the Perigee procedures performed in conjunction with sacrospinous hysteropexy.

Figure 8-10 Anterior compartment transobturator polypropylene mesh is secured to the distal cervix in those who undergo uterine preservation at the time that anterior compartment surgery is performed.

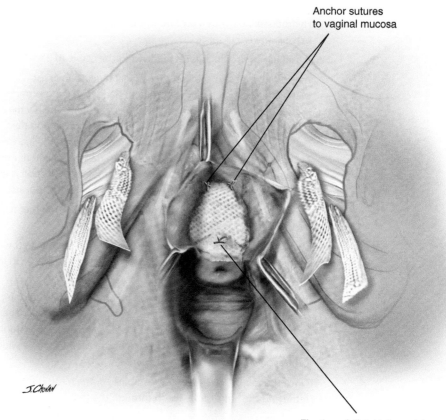

Anchor sutures to vaginal mucosa

Fixation of distal tail mesh to anterior lip of cervix

Case 4: Mesh Augmented Anterior Repair

View: Videos 8-9 and 8-10

The patient is a 73-year-old woman with a body mass index (BMI) of 40; she has complete uterine procidentia and complete eversion of the anterior and posterior vaginal walls. The uterus extends approximately 14 cm beyond the introitus. The patient is referred from an ancillary hospital; she has been in complete urinary retention for a prolonged period and has developed bilateral renal compromise. She is unable to maintain a pessary in place. With extreme difficulty, two double-J ureteral stents are placed to facilitate the drainage of urine with the prolapse down. After medical clearance is obtained, the plan is to proceed with a vaginal hysterectomy, a vaginal vault suspension to the sacrospinous ligament with anterior synthetic mesh augmentation, and a posterior colpoperineorrhaphy.

Procedural Steps

1. Vaginal hysterectomy is performed. (Chapter 4 for details of vaginal hysterectomy for complete uterine procidentia.)

2. Three sutures are passed extraperitoneally through the right coccygeus–sacrospinous ligament (C-SSL) muscle complex, and sutures are brought out through the full thickness of the posterior vaginal wall as previously described and demonstrated for sacrospinous colpopexy.

3. The Elevate Anterior System (American Medical Systems [AMS]) begins similarly to the dissection previously described for trocar-based systems. The procedure starts with

hydrodissection of the anterior vaginal wall with an anesthetic and epinephrine to the level of 1 to 2 cm proximal to the external urethral meatus. A full-thickness vaginal wall incision is made in the midline, cutting into the epithelium and underlying muscularis and into the vesicovaginal space. Metzenbaum scissors are used to sharply dissect the vaginal wall away from the underlying bladder mucosa to create the vesicovaginal space. The dissection is extended laterally to the superior pubic rami, which is best accomplished by keeping the scissors parallel to the vaginal epithelium and pointing toward the ipsilateral shoulder. Once this level of lateral dissection is extended into the paravaginal space, blunt or sharp dissection is used to mobilize completely the bladder and to enter the paravaginal space, which then allows easy access to the ischial spines and C-SSL muscle complex.

4. A previously cut Elevate mesh is then brought into the field and fixed distally at the level of the bladder neck by passing polypropylene anchors into the lateral pelvic sidewall obturator internus muscle using a specially designed needle. The distal edge of the mesh is sutured into the pubocervical fascia with delayed absorbable sutures or into the anterior leaf of the peritoneum in patients with massive prolapse whose peritoneum is open and in patients who are undergoing a specific colpopexy procedure.

5. The Elevate fixation arms are then passed into the C-SSL muscle complex on each side. A specially designed sheath protects the fixating tip, and the needle tip is configured to allow perpendicular insertion into the ligament. The arms are then brought out through a specific opening in the mesh on each side. An adjustment tool is used to push the mesh down onto the fixation arms.

6. Once the mesh has been advanced and the appropriate tension obtained, locking eyelets are used to lock the mesh in place, leaving them in their appropriate position (Figure 8-11).

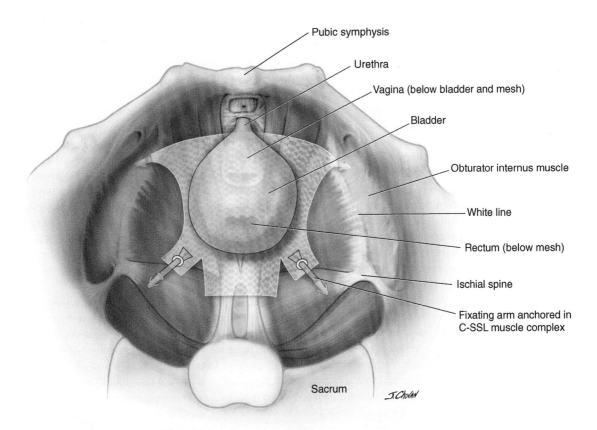

Pubic symphysis

Urethra

Vagina (below bladder and mesh)

Bladder

Obturator internus muscle

White line

Rectum (below mesh)

Ischial spine

Fixating arm anchored in C-SSL muscle complex

Sacrum

J. Chovan

Elevate mesh, anterior placement
(pelvic view from above)

Figure 8-11 The Elevate incisonless mesh (American Medical Systems [AMS]) is bilaterally anchored to the sacrospinous ligament and obturator internus muscle near the distal end of the arcus tendineus fascia pelvis (ATFP).

7. With this particular patient, a significant amount of vagina is excised, leaving adequate vagina to close over the mesh with minimal tension. Interrupted delayed absorbable sutures or a running suture is then used to close the anterior vaginal wall and vaginal apex.

8. The sacrospinous ligament fixation stitches are tied, which elevates the prolapsed apex to be in direct contact with the right C-SSL.

9. Cystoscopic examination is performed to ensure that no inadvertent bladder injury has occurred and that both ureteral orifices with the ureteral stents in place are visualized. If stents were not used, then the surgeon will need to observe a bilateral spill from each ureter to ensure patency.

10. The procedure is completed with a posterior colporrhaphy and extensive perineorrhaphy.

See Videos 8-9 and 8-10 for video demonstrations of a mesh-augmented anterior repair using the Elevate Anterior System with vaginal hysterectomy and in the patient with a recurrent cystocele after a hysterectomy.

Case Discussion

The previous two cases discuss mesh augmentation, which has been beneficial in the experience of the authors of this text in selected settings of large cystoceles and recurrent cystoceles. In the presence of a large cystocele, the potential advantages of mesh placement is twofold; it facilitates anterior vaginal wall support, hopefully providing a more durable long-term success, but it also simplifies the repair and is placed without requiring any type of plication, which tends to standardize the repair. To date, minimal long-term data are available on the Elevate Anterior System. Some surgeons prefer to use a direct access system over trocar-based systems for the theoretical advantages of avoiding the inner thigh and transobturator muscles, as well as possibly decreasing the amount of mesh shrinkage as a result of the lack of arms passed through the obturator membrane. To date, no comparative trials are available to comparing this system with the more traditional trocar-based mesh kits as have been described and discussed in previous cases.

In case 3, the surgeon preferred an armed transobturator mesh using either the Perigee mesh (AMS) or the anterior Prolift mesh (Johnson & Johnson). The Perigee mesh has a RCT with 1-year follow-up attesting to its anatomic superiority to anterior colporrhaphy. (Nguyen, Burchette, 2008) More recently, Altman et al (2011) reported on behalf of the Nordic Transvaginal mesh group, who compared the anterior Prolift (*n* = 189) with anterior colporrhaphy and included those with stage 2 symptomatic cystocele without any need for concomitant prolapse or continence surgery. They reported improved subjective and objective outcomes in the mesh group, and these advantages were offset by longer surgical time and greater blood loss, greater number cystotomy procedures, a greater difficulty emptying the bladder, and inguinal pain in early postoperative phases in the mesh group. No differences in reoperation rates for prolapse were observed in 1 year (1 case in the native tissue repair group), whereas the reoperation rate was higher in the mesh group for urinary stress incontinence and mesh exposure, as well as a possible higher rate for *de novo* dyspareunia. In a small comparative study evaluating Perigee and Prolift, the authors of this text were not able to demonstrate a significant difference between the two products in the management of anterior compartment prolapse, and both continue to be used. More recently, as discussed in case 4, some surgeons prefer the Elevate Anterior System, which is a single-incision mesh kit that does not require trocars.

Clearly in both cases, apical support is required, and hysteropexy and hysterectomy vault suspension are options, depending on patient desires. (This discussion is fully undertaken in Chapter 6.) Routinely, a hysteropexy seems to be the preferred approach; however, in patients with large uterine prolapse, hysterectomy seems to be the preference without any evidence to support this approach. With the information available from Delancey (1993), over 50% of anterior compartment prolapse is caused by apical prolapse. Larson and colleagues (2009) used three-dimensional magnetic resonance imaging (MRI) to superimpose the relative position of the mesh kits anchoring through the ATFP on the vagina. They found that the anterior vagina extended above the superior attachment points in 100% of women at rest and in 73% during the Valsalva maneuver. In addition, the bladder extended below the distal mesh insertion in 82% of women at rest and 100% during the Valsalva maneuver. The mean percentage of anterior vaginal length above superior anchoring sites was 40 at rest (±14%) and 29 during the Valsalva maneuver (±12%). (Larson, Hsu, DeLancey, 2009) In response to the conclusions that the upper vagina lies above and posterior to the suspension points in most women, the authors of this text have, for some time, used the tail of both the Perigee mesh and the Prolift mesh to secure continuous repair between the level 2 anterior mesh repair and level support. This is achieved in hysteropexy by securing the tail to the cervix anteriorly and then, if required, the posterior lip of the cervix to the right sacrospinous ligament, which is fully described in the hysteropexy section (Chapter 4). In women undergoing hysterectomy (if the surgery is performed vaginally) or in women who have had a hysterectomy, the tail of the mesh is secured directly to the right sacrospinous ligament as discussed and demonstrated in the vaginal vault Chapter 7.

Outcomes

In women with large anterior compartment (extending beyond the introitus), anterior colporrhaphy has a higher risk of anterior compartment prolapse as compared to transobturator polypropylene mesh (RR 3.55, 95%; CI 2.29 to 5.51) (Maher et al, 2010) This reduction in anterior compartment prolapse is greater than the benefit achieved with mesh overlay alone (RR 2.14, 95%; CI 1.23 to 3.74). Furthermore, a significantly higher rate of mesh erosions in self-styled meshes is suggested, as compared with commercial kits with Nieminen reporting a 17% rate of mesh erosions at 1 year and a 19% rate at 3 years with self-styled mesh. (Hiltunen et al, 2007; Nieminen et al, 2010) In addition, in a recent retrospective comparison study, the overall mesh erosion rate was 11.3%, a significantly lower 1.4% (1 of 69) erosion rate when using commercial kits versus 23.6% (13 of 55) when using overlay synthetic grafts. (Finamore et al, 2010) More data are required in comparing self-styled meshes with commercially produced kits.

Although this benefit on anterior compartment mesh is established in reduced objective and subjective recurrences, the clinician needs to be cautious and mindful of potential problems associated with the commercial-armed kits as outlined. Most of these trials report anterior compartment prolapse as the objective outcome, which needs to be reconsidered in light of the report that suggests a 46% rate of *de novo* pelvic organ prolapse (POP), stage II or higher, at other sites after an isolated anterior Prolift repair in 150 women. (Withagen, Vierhout, Milani, 2010) In evaluating anterior vaginal meshes, the Cochrane review reported no differences in sexual function using the Pelvic Organ Prolapse/Urinary Incontinence Sexual Questionnaire–short version (PISQ-12) when comparing anterior meshes with anterior colporrhaphy. Interestingly, Altman et al (2011) in a large RCT comparing anterior Prolift and anterior colporrhaphy found *de novo* dyspareunia in 2% of the anterior colporrhaphy group and 7.3% in the mesh group, raising the possibility that many of the papers may be underpowered to detect a real difference in *de novo* dyspareunia rates, if they exist. In a larger multi-center prospective study of 84 women, 1 year after Prolift transvaginal mesh surgery, the overall sexual function scores (PISQ-12) worsened from 15.5 at baseline to 11.7 1 year after surgery (p <0.001). The trend toward deteriorating sexual function scores was similar for anterior, posterior, and total Prolift procedures. An overall worsening of all symptoms was revealed in the behavioral emotive–related and partner-related items, whereas improvements were observed in physical. (Altman et al, 2009) In a recent case control study comparing native tissue repairs (185) to Prolift repairs (138), Fatton and colleagues (2010) demonstrated that the *de novo* dyspareunia rate was 2% in the native tissue repair group, as compared with 16% in the Prolift mesh group (p = 0.04). The overall sexual function PISQ-12 scores significantly improved in the native tissue repair group, as compared with nonsignificant changes after the Prolift procedure.

Although these are early reports, the consistent direction of the deterioration in sexual function in case control studies with the Prolift procedure raises concerns that necessitate greater evaluation.

Rare Presentations

If advanced prolapse is ignored for a prolonged period, the prolapse can become incarcerated, making the management more complex. Several years ago, the authors of this text were asked to examine a patient who was 68 years of age with a long-standing procidentia for which the patient had previously refused treatment. She experienced extreme abdominal and vaginal pain, and a vaginal examination revealed a large procidentia with the bladder completely exteriorized through the urethra (Figure 8-12). The vaginal prolapse was not able to be reduced in the office. An IVP performed (see Figure 8-12, *B*) revealed the ureters completely obstructed and lying outside of the pelvic view, indicating the exteriorized tissue included ureters bilaterally. The gross clubbing of the calyces indicated the longevity of the ureteric obstruction, and her creatinine level was double the upper limit of normal. This woman was brought to the surgical unit and underwent vaginal hysterectomy anterior and posterior repair and sacrospinous colpopexy. With the prolapse reduced and the bladder reduced through the urethra while under general anesthesia, an indwelling catheter was placed for 10 days. On removal of the indwelling catheter, the bladder did not prolapse again; at 2 months, the blood parameters and IVP were completely normal, leading the patient to conclude that she was presented for treatment at the right time!!

A second rare case involved a 78-year-old woman with a long-standing procidentia that was creating significant pain and urinary retention. Over time, the patient was unable to reduce the prolapse manually. On examination in the office, the uterus was nonreducible, and a large firm mass was easily palpable in the anterior vaginal wall (Figure 8-13). The patient was taken to the surgical department where a vaginal hysterectomy was performed. Cystoscopic examination confirmed a large intravesical stone had formed within the nonreducible prolapse. Vaginal cystotomy was necessary to remove the stone. The cystotomy was repaired in two layers using 3.0 chromic sutures, and a native tissue repair of the prolapse was performed. The patient had an eventual return of normal bladder function.

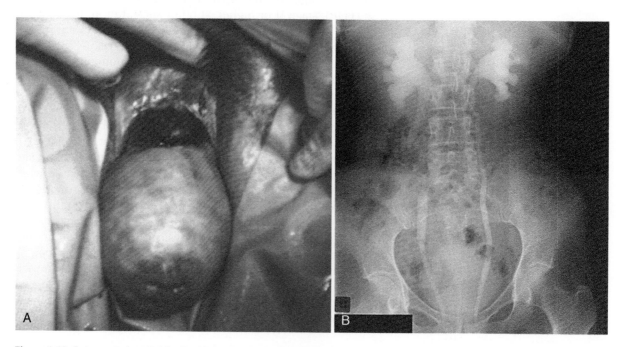

Figure 8-12 A, Large uterine procidentia with exteriorization of the bladder through the urethra is demonstrated. **B,** Intravenous pyelogram (IVP) reveals a gross bilateral hydroureter and clubbing of the renal calyces.

Figure 8-13 A, Large nonreducible uterovaginal prolapse is demonstrated. **B,** Complete eversion of the anterior vaginal wall is visualized with evidence of a firm palpable mass separate from the uterus.

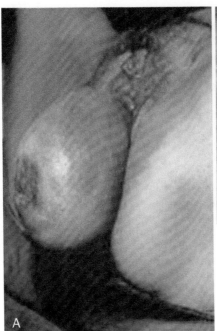

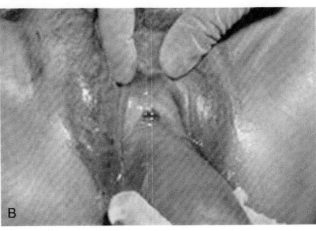

SUMMARY: Important conclusions on anterior compartment prolapse surgery are summarized and outline the authors' approach to a variety of clinical presentations:

- Apical support accounts for up to 50% anterior compartment prolapse and should regularly addressed at POP surgery

- Isolated anterior compartment prolapse: anterior colporrhaphy incorporating anterior cervix

- Moderate anterior compartment prolapse with SUI: retropubic colposuspension with paravaginal repair or anterior colporrhaphy with suburethral tape

- Large or recurrent anterior compartment prolapse with uterine descent: polypropylene mesh with hysteropexy or anterior polypropylene mesh with hysterectomy and tail of mesh to sacrospinous ligament or uterosacral ligaments

- Large anterior compartment prolapse with vault prolapse: sacral colpopexy with paravaginal repair or anterior mesh with tail incorporating sacrospinous or uterosacral ligament

- Large anterior compartment prolapse: part of posthysterectomy prolapse in older and frail women who do not desire sexual function colpocleisis

- Vaginal mesh surgery: ongoing rigorous evaluation required

- Biological grafts to augment anterior compartment: further evaluation required

Suggested Readings

Altman D, Elmér C, Kiilholma P, et al: Sexual dysfunction after trocar-guided transvaginal mesh repair of pelvic organ prolapse, *Obstet Gynecol* 113(1):127–133, 2009.

Altman D, Väyrynen T, Engh ME, et al: Anterior colporrhaphy versus transvaginal mesh for pelvic-organ prolapse, *N Engl J Med* 364(19):1826–1836, 2011.

Brubaker L, Bump RC, Fynes M, et al: Surgery for pelvic organ prolapse, In Abrams P, Cordozo L, Koury S, Wein A, editors: 3rd International Consultation on Incontinence, Paris, 2005, Health Publication Ltd.

Bruce RG, El Galley RE, Galloway NT: Paravaginal defect repair in the treatment of female stress urinary incontinence and cystocele, *Urology* 54(4):647–651, 1999.

Chmielewski L, Walters MD, Weber AM, et al: Reanalysis of a randomized trial of 3 techniques of anterior colporrhaphy using clinically relevant definitions of success, *Am J Obstet Gynecol* 205(1): 69.e1-e8, 2011.

Denman MA, Gregory WT, Boyles SH, et al: Reoperation rate 10 years after surgically managed pelvic organ prolapse and urinary incontinence, *Am J Obstet Gynecol* 198:555.e1-e5, 2008.

DeLancey JO: Anatomy and biomechanics of genital prolapse, *Clinical obstetrics and gynecology* 36(4):897-909, 1993.

Elkins TE, Chesson. RR, Videla F, et al: Transvaginal paravaginal repair. A useful adjunctive procedure at pelvic relaxation surgery, *J Pelvic Surg* 6:11-15, 2000.

Fatton B, Lagrange E, Jacquetin B: Sexual outcome after transvaginal repair of pelvic organ prolapse (POP) with and without mesh: a prospective study of 323 patients, Available at http://www.icsoffice.org/Abstracts/Publish/105/000053.pdf, 2010.

Finamore PS, Echols KT, Hunter K, et al: Risk factors for mesh erosion 3 months following vaginal reconstructive surgery using commercial kits vs. fashioned mesh-augmented vaginal repairs, *Int Urogynecol J* 21(3):285-291, 2010.

Flood CG, Drutz HP, Waja L: Anterior colporrhaphy reinforced with Marlex mesh for the treatment of cystoceles, *Int Urogynecol J Pelvic Floor Dysfunct* 9(4):200-204, 1998.

Grody MHT, Nyirjesy P, Kelley LM, et al: Paraurethral fascial sling urethropexy and vaginal paravaginal defects cystopexy in the correction of urethrovesical prolapse, *Int Urogynecol J Pelvic Floor Dysfunct* 6:80-85, 1995.

Hiltunen R, Nieminen K, Takala T, et al: Low-weight polypropylene mesh for anterior vaginal wall prolapse: a randomized controlled trial, *Obstet Gynecol* 110(2 Pt 2):455-462, 2007.

Hsu Y, Chen L, Summers A, et al: Anterior vaginal wall length and degree of anterior compartment prolapse seen on dynamic MRI, *Int Urogynecol J Pelvic Floor Dysfunct* 19(1):137-142, 2008.

Julian TM: The efficacy of Marlex mesh in the repair of severe, recurrent vaginal prolapse of the anterior midvaginal wall, *Am J Obstet Gynecol* 175(6):1472-1475, 1996.

Kelly HA: Incontinence of urine in women, *Urol Cutaneous Rev* 17:291-293, 1913.

Larson KA, Hsu Y, DeLancey JO: The relationship between superior attachment points for anterior wall mesh operations and the upper vagina using a 3-dimensional magnetic resonance model in women with normal support, *Am J Obstet Gynecol* 200(5):554.e1-e6, 2009.

Macer GA: Transabdominal repair of cystocele, a 20 year experience, compared with the traditional vaginal approach, *Am J Obstet Gynecol* 131(2):203-207, 1978.

Maher C, Feiner B, Baessler K, et al: Surgical management of pelvic organ prolapse in women, *Cochrane Database Syst Rev* 4:CD004014, 2010.

Mallipeddi PK, Steele AC, Kohli N, et al: Anatomic and functional outcome of vaginal paravaginal repair in the correction of anterior vaginal wall prolapse, *Int Urogynecol J Pelvic Floor Dysfunct* 12(2):83-88, 2001.

Nguyen JN, Burchette RJ: Outcome after anterior vaginal prolapse repair: a randomized controlled trial, *Obstet Gynecol* 111(4):891-898, 2008.

Nieminen K, Hiltunen R, Takala T, et al: Outcomes after anterior vaginal wall repair with mesh: a randomized, controlled trial with a 3 year follow-up, *Am J Obstet Gynecol* 203(3):235.e1-e8, 2010.

Olsen AL, Smith VJ, Bergstrom JO, et al: Epidemiology of surgically managed pelvic organ prolapse and urinary incontinence, *Obstet Gynecol* 89(4):501-506, 1997.

Porges RF, Smilen SW: Long-term analysis of the surgical management of pelvic support defects, *Am J Obstet Gynecol* 171(6):1518-1528, 1994.

Richardson AC, Lyon JB, Williams NL: A new look at pelvic relaxation, *Am J Obstet Gynecol* 126:568-573, 1976.

Richardson AC, Edmonds PB, Williams NL: Treatment of stress urinary incontinence due to paravaginal fascial defect, *Obstet Gynecol* 57(3):357-362, 1981.

Sand PK, Koduri S, Lobel RW, et al: Prospective randomized trial of polyglactin 910 mesh to prevent recurrence of cystoceles and rectoceles, *Am J Obstet Gynecol* 184(7):1357-1362, 2001.

Scotti RJ, Garely AD, Greston WM, et al: Paravaginal repair of lateral vaginal wall defects by fixation to the ischial periosteum and obturator membrane, *Am J Obstet Gynecol* 179(6 Pt 1):1436-1445, 1998.

Shull BL, Baden WF: A six-year experience with paravaginal defect repair for stress urinary incontinence, *Am J Obstet Gynecol* 160:1432-1440, 1989.

Shull BL, Benn SJ, Kuehl TJ: Surgical management of prolapse of the anterior vaginal segment: an analysis of support defects, operative morbidity, and anatomical outcome, *Am J Obstet Gynecol* 171:1429-1439, 1994.

Sivaslioglu A, Unlubilgin E, Dolen I: A randomised comparison of polypropelene mesh surgery with site-specific surgery in treatment of cystocele, *Int Urogynecol J Pelvic Floor Dysfunct* 19(4):467-471, 2008.

Stanton SL, Hilton P, Norton C, et al: Clinical and urodynamic effects of anterior colporrhaphy and vaginal hysterectomy for prolapse with and without incontinence, *Br J Obstet Gynaecol* 89(6):459–463, 1982.

Summers A, Winkel LA, Hussain HK, et al: The relationship between anterior and apical compartment support, *Am J Obstet Gynecol* 194(5):1438–1443, 2006.

Vollebregt A, Fischer K, Gietelink D, et al: Primary surgical repair of anterior vaginal prolapse: a randomised trial comparing anatomical and functional outcome between anterior colporrhaphy and trocar-guided transobturator anterior mesh, *BJOG* 118(12):1518–1527, 2011.

Walter S, Olesen KP, Hald T, et al: Urodynamic evaluation after vaginal repair and colposuspension, *Br J Urol* 54(4):377–380, 1982.

Weber AM, Walters MD, Piedmonte MR, et al: Anterior colporrhaphy: a randomized trial of three surgical techniques, *Am J Obstet Gynecol* 185(6):1299–1304, 2001.

White GR: Cystocele, *JAMA* 853:1707–1710, 1909.

White GR: An anatomical operation for the cure of cystocele, *Am J Obstet Dis Women Child* 65:286–290, 1912.

Withagen MI, Vierhout ME, Milani AL: Does trocar-guided tension-free vaginal mesh (Prolift) repair provoke prolapse of the unaffected compartments? *Int Urogynecol J* 21(3):271–278, 2010.

Young SB, Daman JJ, Bony LG: Vaginal paravaginal repair: one-year outcomes, *Am J Obstet Gynecol* 185(6):1360–1366, 2001.

Surgical Correction of Posterior Pelvic Floor Defects

Mickey Karram, MD

 Video Clips online

9-1 Anatomy of the Posterior Vaginal Wall
9-2 Defect-Specific Rectocele Repair
9-3 Rectocele Repair in Conjunction with Repair of Posterior Enterocele

9-4 Rectocele Repair in Conjunction with Repair of Anal Sphincter Repair
9-5 Rectocele and Enterocele Repair Augmented with Biologic Mesh

Posterior pelvic floor defects include a variety of pelvic floor support disorders and anatomic defects of the anal sphincter. These various abnormalities may be asymptomatic, create traditional symptoms of prolapse, or result in a variety of functional arrangements. Posterior vaginal wall prolapse co-exists with anterior or apical prolapse in up to 50% of patients. Various types of posterior wall prolapse include a posterior enterocele, rectocele, sigmoidocele, and perineal descent (Figure 9-1). Although these various defects can occur in isolation, they commonly occur in combination. Defects in the external anal sphincter, which anatomically make up a significant portion of the perineum, can contribute to a gapping perineum and may also contribute to incontinence of either gas, liquid, or solid stool.

A *rectocele* is best defined as an anterior protrusion of the rectal wall into the posterior vaginal wall. The rectovaginal space is occupied by areolar tissue and allows the vagina and the rectum to function independently of each other. Although many theories and anatomic descriptions describe the support of the posterior vaginal wall, it is probably best described as a complex interaction between the connective tissue support and muscular support of the pelvic floor that maintains the integrity of the vaginal tube.

An *enterocele* is a hernia in which the peritoneum and abdominal contents displace the vagina and may even be in contact with vaginal mucosa. The normal intervening endopelvic fascia is deficient or absent, and small bowel fills the hernia sac. Generally, enteroceles have been divided into four types: congenital, traction, pulsion, and iatrogenic. Factors that may predispose a woman to the development of congenital enteroceles include neurologic disorders such as spina bifida and connective tissue disorders. Traction enteroceles occur secondary to uterovaginal prolapse, and pulsion enteroceles are the result of prolonged increases in intraabdominal pressure. Iatrogenic enteroceles occur after surgical procedures that elevate the normally horizontal vaginal axis in a vertical direction, such as a colposuspension for stress incontinence or after hysterectomy if the vaginal cuff and cul-de-sac are not appropriately managed. Clinically, enteroceles are best classified based on their anatomic location. Apical enteroceles herniate through the apex of the vagina, posterior enteroceles herniate posteriorly to the vaginal apex, and anterior enteroceles herniate anterior to the vaginal apex (Figure 9-2).

The descent of the sigmoid colon into the lower pelvic cavity, leading to mechanical obstruction of the rectum, is a *sigmoidocele.*

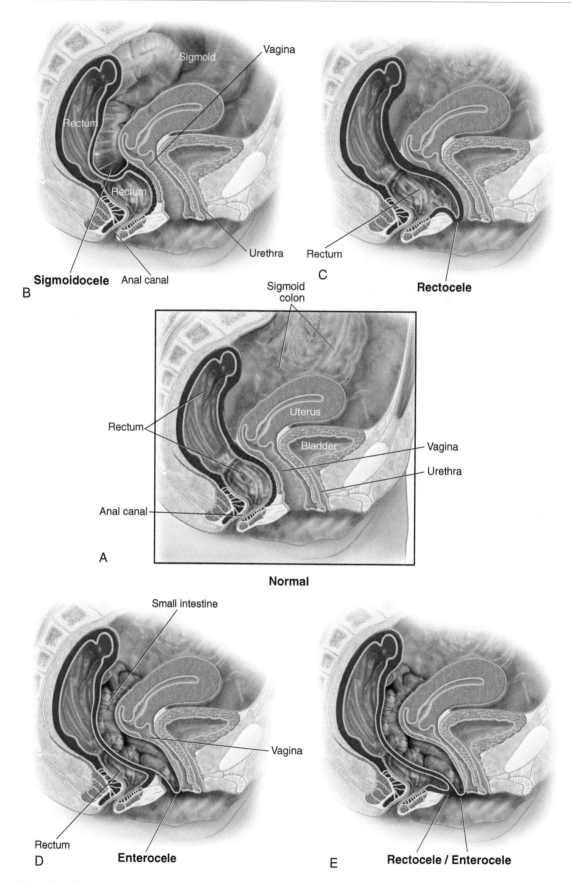

Figure 9-1 Different types of posterior pelvic floor prolapse. **A,** Normal anatomy. **B,** Sigmoidocele, a rare type of prolapse that mimics a high rectocele or enterocele. **C,** Rectocele in isolation. **D,** Enterocele in isolation. **E,** Combined rectocele and enterocele.

(From Hull TL: Posterior pelvic floor abnormalities. In Karram M, editor: Female pelvic surgery video atlas series. Philadelphia, 2011, Elsevier.)

Figure 9-2 Cross-section of pelvic floor shows various anatomic locations of enteroceles. **A,** Anterior enterocele—defect in the pubocervical fascia near its attachment to the vaginal apex. The peritoneal sac with its contents protrudes anterior to the vaginal cuff. **B,** Apical enterocele—defect at the vaginal apex; the peritoneal sac protrudes between the pubocervical fascia anterior and the rectovaginal fascia posterior. **C,** Posterior enterocele—defect posterior to the vaginal cuff. The peritoneal sac protrudes through the defect in rectovaginal fascia, posterior to the vaginal cuff.

(Modified from Walters MD, Karram MM, editors: Urogynecology and reconstructive pelvic surgery, *ed 3, Philadelphia, 2007, Elsevier.)*

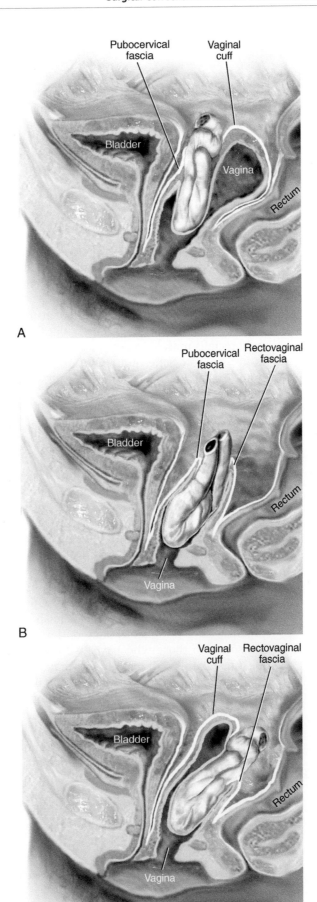

DeLancey (1999) divided the connective tissue support of the vagina into three levels. All three levels of support should be evaluated and addressed during the surgical management of the posterior vaginal wall. Level I support is the uppermost or apical portion of the posterior vaginal wall and is suspended and supported primarily by the cardinal and uterosacral ligaments. Level II support includes the support of the middle half of the vagina, and this support is provided by the endopelvic fascia attaching the lateral posterior vaginal wall to the aponeurosis of the levator ani muscle on the pelvic side wall. The perineal body includes interlacing muscle fibers of the bulbocavernosus, transverse perineal, and external anal sphincter muscles. Anteriorly, the perineum is attached to the vaginal epithelium and muscularis of the posterior vaginal wall. Laterally, it is attached to the ischiopubic ramus through the transverse perineal muscles and the perineal membrane. The perineal body is described as extending cranially on the posterior vaginal wall to approximately 2 to 3 centimeters proximal to the hymenal ring. This dense fused level of support is what DeLancey has described as level III support. Posterior to the perineal body includes the anterior portion of the external anal sphincter and its attachment to the longitudinal fibrous sheet of the internal anal sphincter (Figure 9-3). **(See Video 9-1, "Anatomy of the Posterior Vaginal Wall."**)

Although no significant causes can be found to explain prolapse and specifically posterior vaginal wall prolapse, one contributing factor relates to the state of the puborectalis muscle in general. In a woman with an intact pelvic floor, the puborectalis is in a chronic state of contraction; this contraction closes the vaginal canal, and the anterior and posterior vaginal walls are in direct opposition. With defecation, the increased pressure placed on the posterior vaginal wall is equalibrated by the opposing anterior vaginal wall, and minimal stress is placed on the endopelvic fascia attachments. If muscular or neurologic damage has occurred to the puborectalis, then the levator hiatus widens and the vaginal canal opens. The increased rectal pressure and distention associated with defecation places a strain on the endopelvic fascial attachments, and the fibromuscularis of the posterior vaginal wall can result in a rectocele and perineal descent. Other factors that can contribute to the development of posterior pelvic floor abnormalities (whether anatomic, functional, or both) include damage to the support of the posterior vaginal wall at the time of vaginal delivery, as well as conditions that create chronic strain and constipation. As previously mentioned, alterations of the axis of the vagina may increase the forces placed on the connective tissue support. For example, historically, over elevation of the anterior vaginal wall with a retropubic urethropexy or needle suspension procedure has resulted in significant rates of posterior vaginal wall prolapse in the form of enteroceles and rectoceles. More recently, patients who have had mesh-augmented repair of an anterior vaginal wall prolapse have a higher chance of developing posterior vaginal wall prolapse, in comparison with those who have had a native tissue repair of the anterior vaginal wall. Most likely, this is due to the fact that abdominal pressure transmission will be directed in its entirety to the weakest segment of the pelvic floor. It would seem that augmenting one segment of the pelvic floor may create a significant discrepancy in support that leads to prolapse of the opposite segment.

Patients with posterior vaginal prolapse may be totally asymptomatic or may have a variety of anatomic and functional complaints. In general, before surgical correction, testing should be undertaken that might help the surgeon truly determine whether anatomic correction will result in symptomatic relief of the patient's complaints. This chapter discusses a variety of techniques used to correct posterior vaginal wall prolapse and perineal defects. (The history, physical examination, and staging of posterior vaginal wall prolapse are discussed in Chapter 3.)

Preoperative Considerations before Surgical Repair

Ellerkmann and colleagues (2001) reported that 25% to 67% of patients with pelvic organ prolapse admit to symptoms of defecatory dysfunction. These symptoms include straining to have a bowel movement, having to splint to facilitate expulsion of stool,

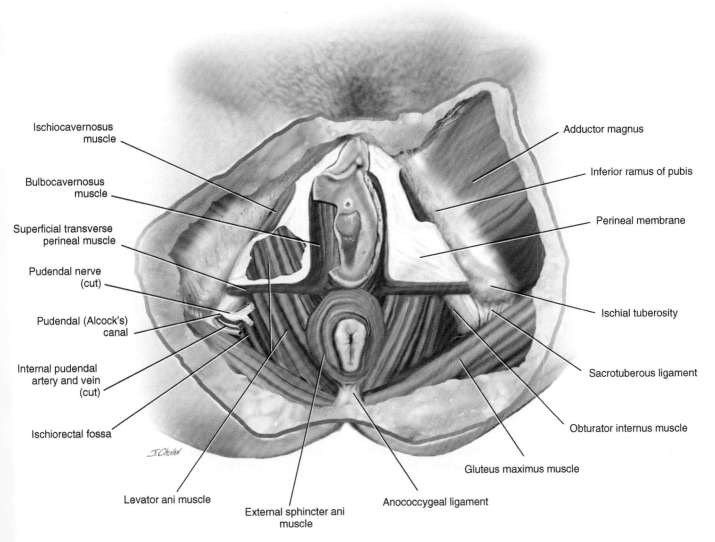

Ischiocavernosus muscle

Bulbocavernosus muscle

Superficial transverse perineal muscle

Pudendal nerve (cut)

Pudendal (Alcock's) canal

Internal pudendal artery and vein (cut)

Ischiorectal fossa

Levator ani muscle

External sphincter ani muscle

Anococcygeal ligament

Gluteus maximus muscle

Obturator internus muscle

Sacrotuberous ligament

Ischial tuberosity

Perineal membrane

Inferior ramus of pubis

Adductor magnus

Figure 9-3 The muscles forming the pelvic floor are visualized. The crural area is prominently seen and felt by the adductor longus muscle. The bulbocavernosus muscle is immediately lateral to the outer wall of the vagina. The ischiocavernosus lies along the margin of the pubic ramus. A tough connective tissue structure called the *perineal membrane* lies between these muscles. Blending into and deep to the bulbocavernosus muscle and external sphincter and muscle is the levator ani muscle. The obturator internus muscle lies between the levator ani and the ramus of the ischium.

(From Baggish MS, Karram MM, editors: Atlas of pelvic anatomy and gynecologic surgery, *ed 3, St Louis, 2011, Elsevier.)*

dyschezia, chronic constipation, and occasional fecal incontinence. Patients may also complain of symptoms related to sexual function. Patients who have an anatomic defect with primarily functional complaints must be thoroughly evaluated and consented before undergoing a surgical procedure, because the correlation between correcting the defect and restoring the functional problems is at times unpredictable. A physical examination should entail a close inspection and assessment of the degree of prolapse, the state of the perineum, the total vaginal length, and the extent and size of the genital or levator hiatus. A rectal examination is performed to further assess the presence and position of a rectocele, as well as help differentiate a rectocele from an enterocele. Inspection and examination of the anal area is also indicated with one finger in the rectum and another in the vagina. A sliding posterior enterocele may be palpated as prolapsed loops of small bowel will become apparent between the intervening tissues of the rectovaginal septum.

At times, further objective assessment of the posterior vaginal wall with either radiographic studies or physiologic studies will help the surgeon determine the potential benefit of surgical intervention. These studies are indicated in patients who have significant bowel symptoms, rather than those patients who have anatomic defects with complaints primarily of prolapse. The main radiologic studies that are used for posterior pelvic floor abnormalities include defecating proctography and dynamic magnetic resonance imaging (MRI). In addition, these studies help rule out other anatomic abnormalities that could be contributing to the patient's symptoms, including sigmoidoceles, anorectal intussusception rectal prolapse, and perineal descent, which can all contribute to the development of symptoms of defecatory dysfunction. The authors prefer to use defecating video proctography to help evaluate the dynamics of evacuation by visualizing the rectum after filling it with liquid barium and determining the extent of the rectocele fluoroscopically. Anal ultrasound is the preferred method for assessing the anal sphincter muscles. Physiologic tests have included anal manometry, electromyography, pudendal nerve terminal motor latency studies, and colonic transit time studies. Except for the transit time studies, the other physiologic studies are only indicated in patients who have significant fecal incontinence; these studies are of minimal clinical use in the patient with posterior pelvic wall prolapse with symptoms of outlet obstruction. The colonic transit time study has been shown to be a good predictor regarding the resolution of difficult evacuation in patients with rectoceles. This study involves serial x-ray examinations of the abdomen used to determine the movement of radiopaque markers after ingesting Sitzmarks capsules. This study may also be helpful as part of the routine preoperative evaluation of patients with rectoceles.

Dynamic MRI provides high-quality images of the pelvic soft tissues and viscera. MRI is noninvasive and does not require ionizing radiation or significant patient preparation. However, poor correlation exists between MRI grading of prolapse and clinical staging. At this time, a standardized method of establishing a radiologic diagnosis of the rectocele is lacking. Clinical examination has good sensitivity for detecting rectoceles, and most enteroceles should be intraoperatively identified during dissection of the upper portion of the posterior vaginal wall. Therefore radiographic confirmation of the presence or absence of posterior vaginal wall prolapse is not worthwhile. Although defecatory dysfunction is common in women with prolapse, the extent of the prolapse does not necessarily correlate with the extent of the bowel symptoms. If the woman's primary complaint is defecatory dysfunction or fecal incontinence and not a bulge, then surgical correction of the rectocele or perineal defect may not correct her symptoms. Specific ancillary testing is then pursued on the basis of the woman's complaints, with the goal of identifying appropriate surgical candidates.

Surgical Management of Posterior Compartment Defects

The surgical indications for posterior vaginal wall prolapse are controversial. Most surgeons advocate operative repair if the prolapse is large, if a rectocele fails to empty on defecography, or if it is clinically associated with frequent vaginal or perineal manipulation by the patient for satisfactory evacuation. Rectocele repair with distal levatorplasty and perineoplasty is also commonly performed in conjunction with repairs of other segments of the pelvic floor or with obliterative procedures to decrease the size of the genital hiatus.

This chapter addresses a variety of different surgical techniques that have been used to correct posterior pelvic organ prolapse. Although the majority of the discussion involves rectocele repair, a discussion of patients with perineal defects, defects of the anal sphincter, and co-existent enteroceles and sigmoidoceles is also included. The goal of these techniques should be to reconstruct the entire posterior vaginal wall as needed from the apex to and including the perineum. The goal of all posterior repair procedures should be to ultimately create a perpendicular relationship between the posterior vaginal wall and the perineum. These procedures should be performed without creating vaginal bands or constrictions but, at the same time, appropriately decreasing the caliber of the genital hiatus if necessary. Other pelvic floor defects, if present, should also be addressed in the same setting.

The published literature continues to classify rectocele repairs into what has been termed as the *traditional technique*, which implies that the repair has been supplemented with a levator ani muscle plication in the midline, or a site-specific technique, which implies that discrete defects in the rectovaginal fascia are identified and repaired and that no levator plication is performed. To date, no studies have addressed how often a posterior enterocele and or sigmoidocele co-exist with a rectocele or how the presence of these defects impacts ultimate surgical outcomes. Based on the current understanding of the anatomy of the posterior vaginal wall and perineum, defect-specific repairs clearly involve plication of the fibromuscular layer of the posterior vaginal wall. Based on the initial level of dissection, this tissue may be found on the anterior wall of the rectum or may have to be mobilized off the vaginal epithelium to allow an appropriate tension-free plication. In patients with advanced prolapse and a widened genital hiatus, the only way to address the gaping vagina is to perform a distal levatorplasty. In the author's opinion, future surgical studies assessing the outcomes of prolapse repair involving the posterior vaginal wall should take into consideration these points and realize that these procedures are not mutually exclusive; a combination of the techniques, especially in cases of advanced prolapse, is commonly required. Other types of repair that have been reported include transanal repairs, transperineal mesh (biologic or synthetic) augmented repairs, and abdominal sacral colpopexy in which the mesh attachment is extended down to the distal portion of the posterior vaginal wall and/or perineum. The author has also observed that aggressive reattachment of the uppermost portion of the full thickness of the posterior vaginal wall (level I support) to the uterosacral ligament provides significant support to the posterior vaginal wall in patients with high rectoceles or rectoceles in conjunction with a posterior enterocele (Figure 9-4).

Technique for Rectocele Repair and Perineoplasty

1. The patient is placed in the lithotomy position in high leg stirrups, and the vagina is sterilely prepared and draped. A catheter is placed to empty the bladder. A pelvic examination under anesthesia, including a careful rectovaginal examination, is performed. The thickness and laxity of the posterior vaginal wall and rectovaginal septum is palpated and closely observed, including how much displacement of the rectal wall protrudes toward the vagina with a palpating finger. The wideness of the levator hiatus and the quality of the levator muscles are bilaterally estimated; the perineal body, not only its length from the posterior fourchette to anus but its thickness, is also palpated. Sometimes a distal perineal rectocele can be quite symptomatic and is only palpable when the rectal finger is hooked backward toward the surgeon during a rectovaginal examination. Because one of the complications of rectocele repair is overzealous fibromuscular or levator plication resulting in vaginal constriction and dyspareunia, the desired caliber of the vagina along its length and especially near the introitus at the hymenal ring is carefully estimated.

2. Two Allis clamps are placed at the posterior fourchette at approximately 5 and 7 o'clock and are gently pulled downward to examine the entire posterior vaginal wall and to again estimate the amount of gaping of the introitus. A dilute hemostatic solution, such as 0.5% Lidocaine with 1:200,000 epinephrine, is injected into the perineum and rectovaginal space. A Lone Star retractor is sometimes useful to help visualize the entire vagina and aid in retraction during a rectocele repair.

3. Some surgeons make a V or diamond incision in the perineum to resect the redundant tissue, and others simply make a midline incision. The authors prefer to excise a diamond-shaped piece of perineal and vaginal skin, based on the desired caliber of the vagina and introitus (Figure 9-5). Once this tissue is excised, Allis clamps are used to grasp the edges of the vaginal epithelium. The author perfers to perform this dissection and the entire repair with a finger in the rectum.

4. The Allis clamps help retract the incised vaginal wall by lifting it. The index finger of the nondominant hand of the surgeon is in the rectum to apply countertraction against the elevated vaginal wall. The rectovaginal space is sharply incised using scissors until the entire vagina is dissected off the rectum to the levator ani muscles,

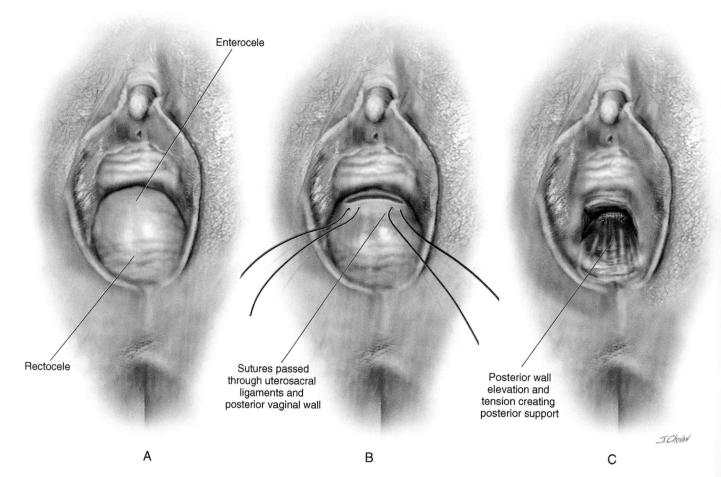

Enterocele

Rectocele

Sutures passed
through uterosacral
ligaments and
posterior vaginal wall

Posterior wall
elevation and
tension creating
posterior support

A   B   C

Figure 9-4 A, Posterior vaginal wall defect, secondary to an enterocele and rectocele, **B,** After entry into the enterocele sac, intraperitoneal suspension sutures are broug
out through the full thickness of the vaginal wall at the level of the apex. **C,** Tying these sutures after the closure of the vaginal incision at the apex does not only result ir
an increase in vaginal length, but it also contributes to the overall support of the entire posterior vaginal wall.

(From Baggish MS, Karram MM, editors: Atlas of pelvic anatomy and gynecologic surgery, *ed 3, St Louis, 2011, Elsevier.)*

which is done bilaterally and proximally; the rectum is separated off the vagina toward the vaginal apex. Once the dissection extends beyond the extraperitoneal portion of the rectum, the rectovaginal space is entered. This is an avascular pre-peritoneal space that allows access to the peritoneum over the cul-de-sac. At times an enterocele can be in the rectovaginal space over the rectocele; consequently, the surgeon should inspect for this and, if an enterocele is identified, correct it (Figure 9-6) The reader is referred to the section, "Technique for Enterocele Repair" on page 150 for a more detailed description. Likewise, if apical prolapse exists, then a sacrospinous ligament or uterosacral colpopexy can be performed before the rectocele repair is completed.

5. A series of sutures are progressively placed bilaterally through the fibromuscular tissue to reduce the rectocele. The vagina should be examined after every two or three sutures to ensure that the posterior vaginal wall is smooth and not becoming too tight during the repair. In addition, irregularities in the posterior vaginal wall from sutures placed at slightly different levels may result in dyspareunia; the offending sutures should be removed and replaced to ensure that the posterior vaginal wall repair is smooth. The repair is begun proximally and extends in a distal direction. The author prefers to perform a two-layered plication when possible (see Figure 9-6).

6. Mixing a partial fibromuscular plication with areas of site-specific defect repair is acceptable, especially in the distal posterior vaginal wall. The surgeon may note a

Figure 9-5 A diamond-shaped piece of perineal and vaginal skin is excised on the basis of the desired caliber of the vagina and introitus.

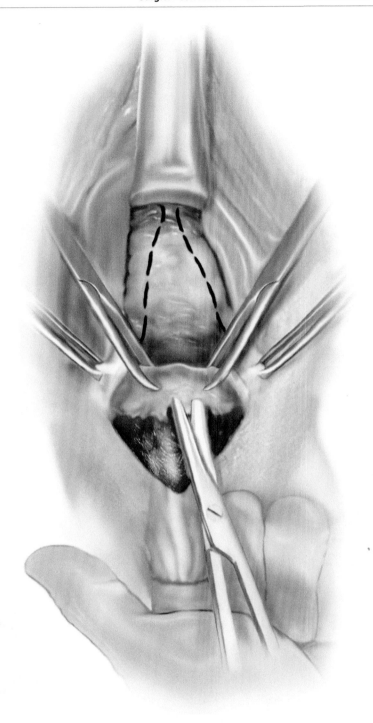

defect in the midline, right, left, or at the perineal body and may be able to identify edges of the fibromuscular tissue or rectovaginal septum. In this case, sutures are placed to repair the defect and even to connect the perineal body to the rectovaginal septum. Performing the repair with a finger in the rectum facilitates the placement of the stitches (Figure 9-7).

7. If necessary, a perineorrhaphy is then performed to help thicken the perineum, both in the craniocaudal direction and in the anteroposterior direction. A rectovaginal examination verifies whether the rectocele has been completely corrected and whether sutures or lacerations are no longer present in the rectal mucosa. The surgeon must be careful not to constrict the hymenal ring too much, which is a frequent cause of entry dyspareunia.

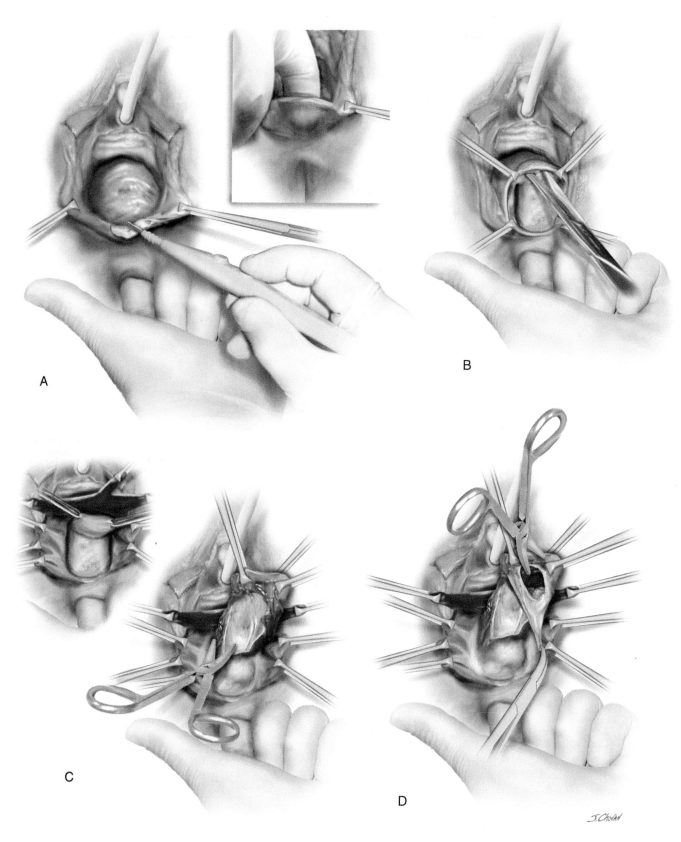

Figure 9-6 Repair of posterior vaginal wall prolapse, including the repair of a rectocele and a posterior enterocele, and perineoplasty. **A,** Built-up perineal skin is incised in the midline. **B,** With a finger in the rectum, sharp dissection is used to mobilize the anterior wall of the rectum off the posterior vaginal wall. **C,** The enterocele sac is mobilized off the anterior wall of the rectum. **D,** Sharp dissection is used to enter the enterocele sac.

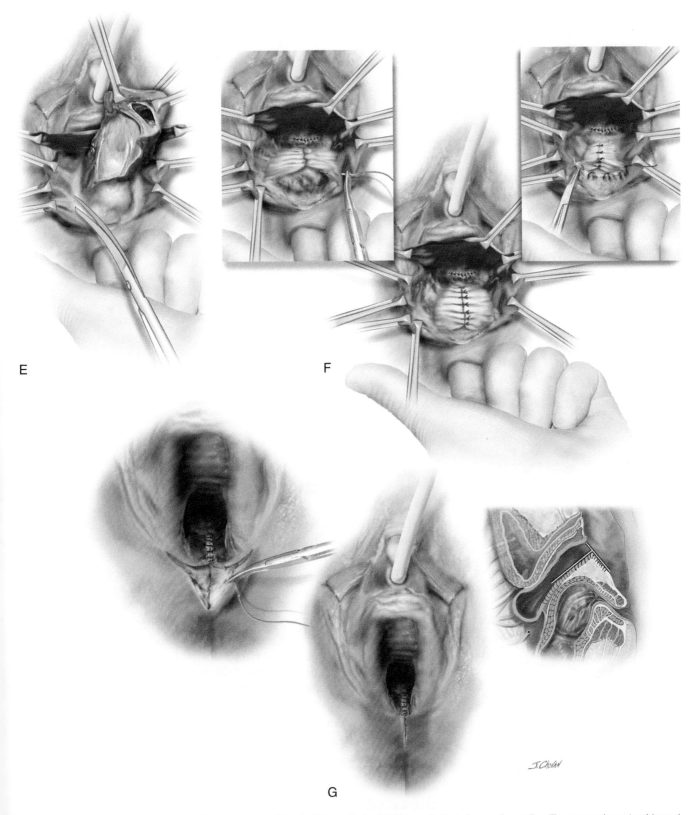

E

F

G

Figure 9-6, cont'd. E, Fibromuscular layer of the vagina is mobilized off the vaginal epithelium and plicated across the midline. The enterocele sac is addressed. **F,** A second layer is mobilized and plicated across the midline. **G,** Perineoplasty is performed; the perpendicular relationship between posterior vaginal wall and perineum is noted.

Figure 9-7 With a finger in the rectum, discrete defects in the fibromuscular layer over the rectum are identified.

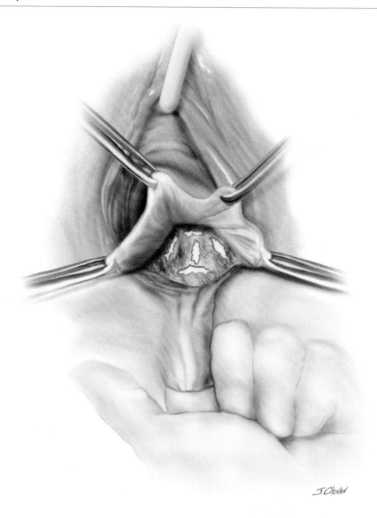

8. The rectovaginal space is carefully visualized for all bleeding vessels that are appropriately cauterized. The rectovaginal space is irrigated, and closure of the posterior vagina is started with a fine running or interrupted delayed absorbable suture. Sometimes, some redundant vaginal wall should be trimmed; however, care should be taken not to over trim and constrict the vagina. The sutures to the hymen are locked, and then the perineorrhaphy incision is closed with simple running or interrupted sutures.

9. No studies have indicated the best type of sutures for rectocele repair. A reasonable choice is a delayed absorbable suture, such as 2.0 Vicryl for the fibromuscular plication of the rectum and the reconstruction of the perineal body; 3.0 Vicryl can be used for closing the posterior vaginal wall and perineal skin.

10. Vaginal packing is reasonable to help decrease the incidence of rectovaginal septum hematoma, but it is not mandatory.

Technique for Enterocele Repair

Patients rarely have an isolated enterocele; usually, concurrent vaginal vault suspension with or without anterior and posterior repair is often necessary. The enterocele sac is usually visualized or digitally identified as a sac or peritoneum separate and distinct from the walls of the bladder or rectum. Surgical repair of an enterocele can be performed vaginally or abdominally. Currently, no data compare the various types of repair. The approach and type of procedure performed depends on the surgeon's preference and whether co-eminent vaginal or abdominal pathologic abnormalities exist. Vaginal surgical techniques described are for traditional vaginal enterocele repair.

(The McCall culdoplasty is described in Chapter 4.) Abdominal approaches discussed include the Moschcowitz and Halban procedures, as well as abdominal uterosacral ligament plication. The technique of vaginal repair of an apical or posterior enterocele follows:

1. A midline vaginal incision is made over the most prominent portion of the suspected enterocele sac. If a rectocele is suspected, then the dissection can be either extended to the perineum or started at the perineum and extended in a cephalad direction. The goal is to open the posterior vaginal wall and dissect the anterior wall of the rectum from the enterocele sac. The dissection should be extended laterally to the median margins of the levator ani muscles.

2. Distinguishing the enterocele sac from the anterior wall of the rectum is facilitated by the use of a rectal finger allowing dissection of the enterocele sac off the anterior wall off the rectum. At times, distinguishing the enterocele sac from a large cystocele may prove difficult. In this situation, placing a probe in the bladder or transilluminating with a cystoscope may be helpful.

3. After the enterocele sac has been dissected away from the vagina, rectum, and bladder, traction is placed on it with two Allis clamps; the sac is palpated to ensure that a small bowel is not adherent to the sac. The enterocele sac is then sharply entered, and the peritoneal cavity is digitally explored to again ensure that no small bowel or omental adhesions are present. If adhesions are encountered, then the goal is to dissect them back to at least the level of the neck of the hernia.

4. Unless an intraperitoneal suspension is to be performed such as a uterosacral suspension, the enterocele sac should be closed using two or three circumferential nonabsorbable purse-string sutures. The cardinal uterosacral ligaments are incorporated into these purse-string sutures. Care should be taken to avoid including the peritoneum in the lateral pelvic side wall to avoid any kink to the ureters. Once all sutures are placed, they are tied in sequence (Figure 9-8).

5. Posterior colporrhaphy and vaginal vault suspension are performed as indicated.

Technique for Abdominal Enterocele Repair

Three techniques of abdominal enterocele repair have been described—the Moschcowitz and Halban procedures and the uterosacral ligament plication.

1. The Moschcowitz procedure is performed by placing concentric purse-string sutures around the cul-de-sac to include the posterior vaginal wall, the right pelvic side wall, the serosa of the sigmoid, and the left pelvic side wall. The initial suture is placed at the base of the cul-de-sac. Usually, three or four sutures completely obliterate the cul-de-sac. The purse-string sutures are tied to ensure that no small defects remain that could entrap small bowel or lead to enterocele recurrence. Care should be taken not to include the ureters in the purse-string sutures or to allow the ureter to be kinked medially when tying the sutures.

2. Halban described a technique to obliterate the cul-de-sac using sutures placed sagittally between the uterosacral ligaments. Four or five sutures are placed sequentially in a longitudinal fashion through the serosa of the sigmoid, into the deep peritoneum of the cul-de-sac, and up the posterior vaginal wall. The sutures are tied, obliterating the cul-de-sac.

3. Transverse plication of the uterosacral ligaments can be used to obliterate the cul-de-sac. Three to five sutures are placed into the medial portion of one uterosacral ligament, into the back wall of the vagina, and into the medial portion of the opposite uterosacral ligament. The lowest suture incorporates the anterior rectal serosa to bring the rectum adjacent to the uterosacral ligaments and vagina. Care must be taken to avoid entrapment or kinking of the ureters. Relaxing incisions can be made in the peritoneum lateral to the uterosacral ligaments to release the ureters, if necessary. Figure 9-9 illustrates these various techniques for the abdominal repair of an enterocele.

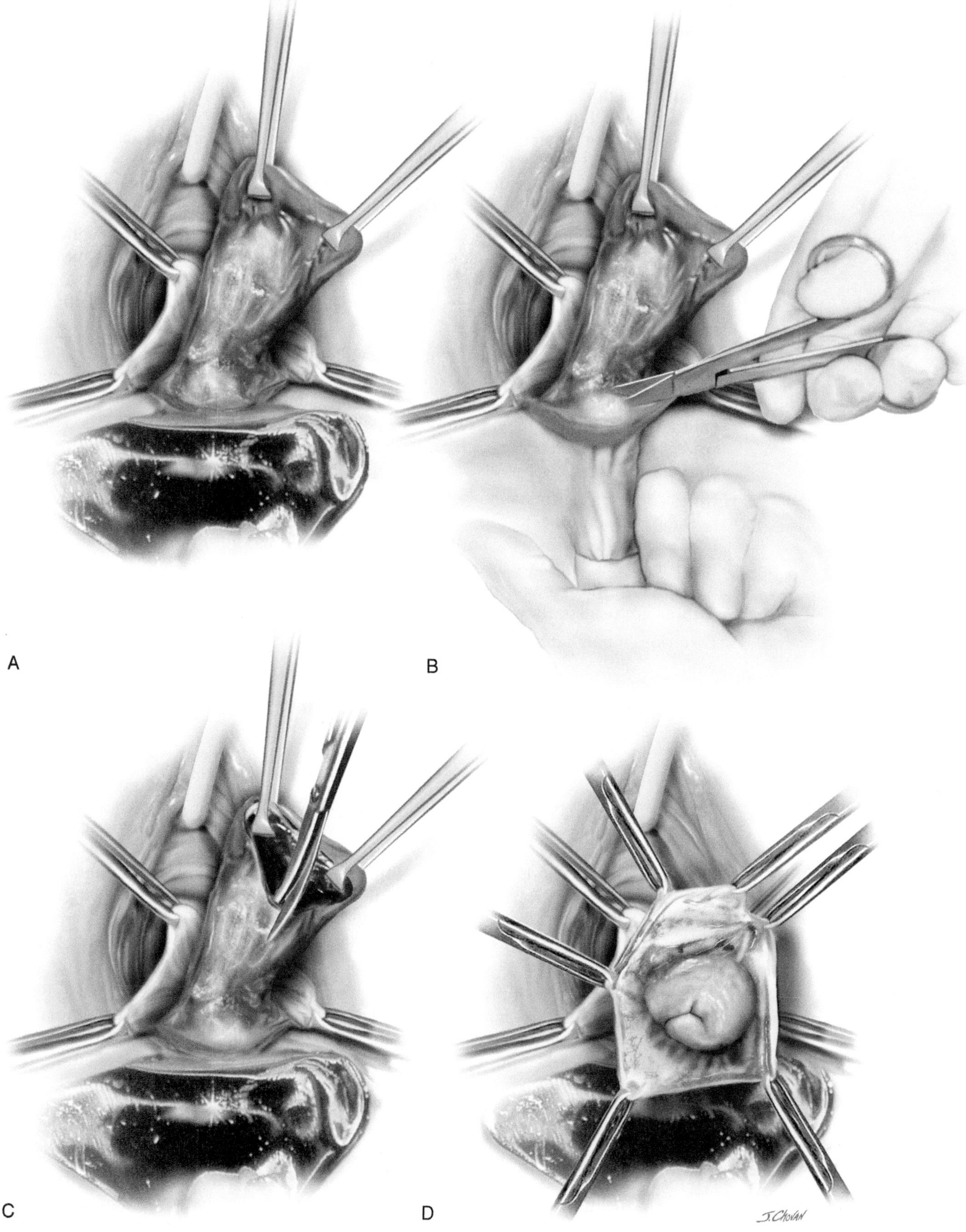

Figure 9-8 Dissection and vaginal repair of the enterocele. **A,** The enterocele sac has been completely mobilized off the vaginal epithelium. **B,** A finger in the rectum facilitates sharp dissection of the enterocele sac off the anterior wall of the rectum. **C,** The enterocele sac is sharply entered. **D,** The peritoneum has been excised, and the cul-de-sac is exposed.

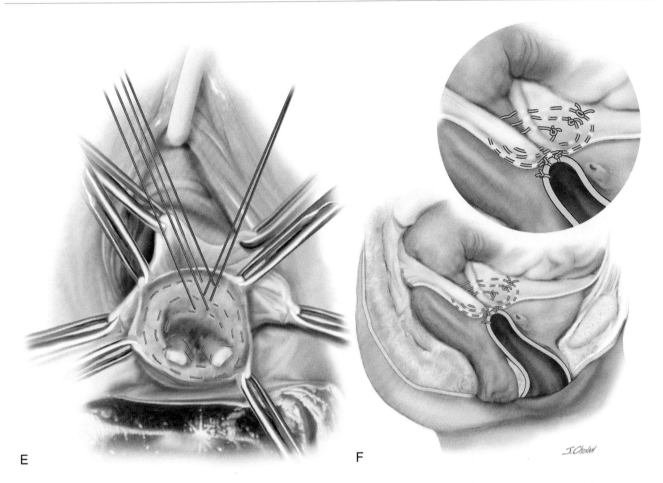

E

F

Figure 9-8, cont'd. E, A series of purse-string sutures incorporating the distal ends of the uterosacral ligaments is placed to close the defect at its neck. **F,** The vaginal apex is attached to the plicated uterosacral ligaments.

(Modified from Walters MD, Karram MM, editors: Urogynecology and reconstructive pelvic surgery, *ed 3, Philadelphia, 2007, Elsevier.)*

Technique for Anal Sphincter Repair

At times, patients will have posterior vaginal wall prolapse and fecal incontinence. When a defect in the sphincteric muscle complex is identified and testing reveals that it is the major factor contributing to the patient's incontinence, a reapproximation of the sphincter should improve the condition. The following is a description of how to perform a sphincteroplasty repair for fecal incontinence.

1. The author of this chapter prefers to perform this repair with a finger in the rectum. An initial inverted U incision is made above the anal opening from the 9- to the 12- to the 3-o'clock position, followed by a midline incision extending up the remainder of the perineum and into the vagina.

2. The mucosa of the vagina is separated from the anterior wall of the rectum sufficiently laterally and superiorly to provide access to the retracted muscles. In addition, the dissection should extend almost to the level of the ischiorectal fossa because most of these patients have a attenuated perineum, and a perineorrhaphy will be performed in conjunction with the anal sphincter repair.

3. Lateral dissection is performed until the ends of the sphincters can be identified. Many times, using a nerve simulator or a low-power cautery to identify viable muscle is helpful; frequently the viable muscle will be surrounded by scar tissue. The author prefers to divide the scar in the middle, leaving the two ends of the sphincter with the scar attached. Dividing the scar, not trimming it, from the ends of the sphincter is important because it will provide tensile strength when the repair is done. The sphincter ends are sufficiently mobilized to allow overlapping of the muscle and are

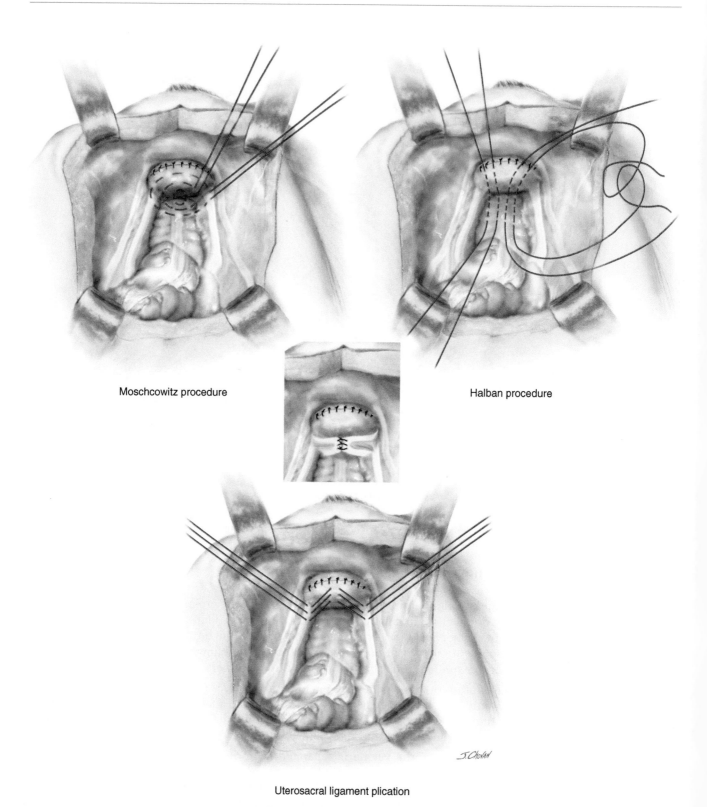

Moschcowitz procedure

Halban procedure

Uterosacral ligament plication

Figure 9-9 Techniques of enterocele repair via the abdominal route: Moschcowitz procedure, Halban procedure, and uterosacral ligament placation.

(Modified from Walters MD, Karram MM, editors: Urogynecology and reconstructive pelvic surgery, *ed 3, Philadelphia, 2007, Elsevier.)*

grasped with the Allis clamps. Numerous mattress sutures are placed through the entire length of the sphincter on each side. Approximately six sutures (three on each side) are used. Mattress-type sutures are used to overlap the edges of the sphincter. During the repair, irrigation of the wound is carried out with an antibiotic solution (Figure 9-10).

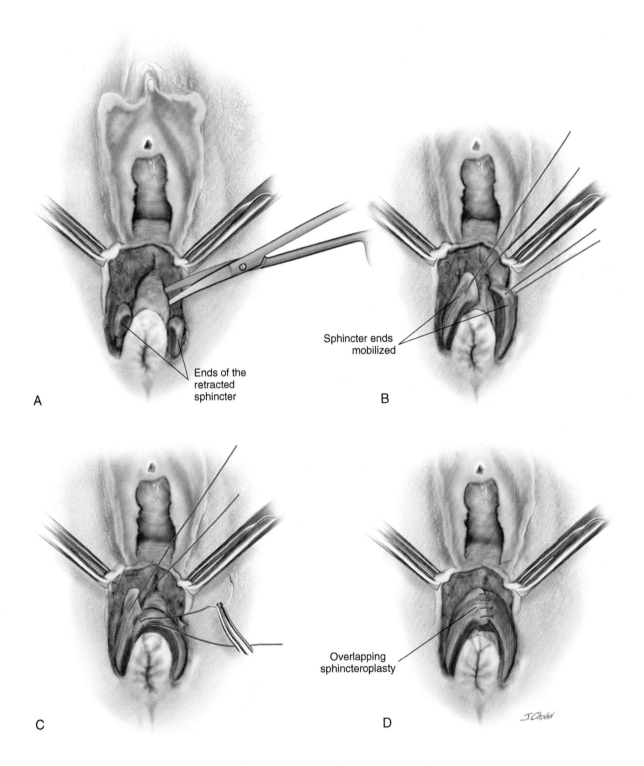

A

Ends of the
retracted
sphincter

B

Sphincter ends
mobilized

C

D

Overlapping
sphincteroplasty

J. Chovan

Figure 9-10 Technique for overlapping sphincteroplasty.

4. If the ends of the anal sphincter are significantly retracted, then performing an overlapping sphincteroplasty becomes impossible. This is commonly observed when a complete breakdown of a third- or fourth-degree episiotomy repair occurs; an end-to-end sphincteroplasty with the incorporation of the internal anal sphincter is then performed (Figure 9-11).

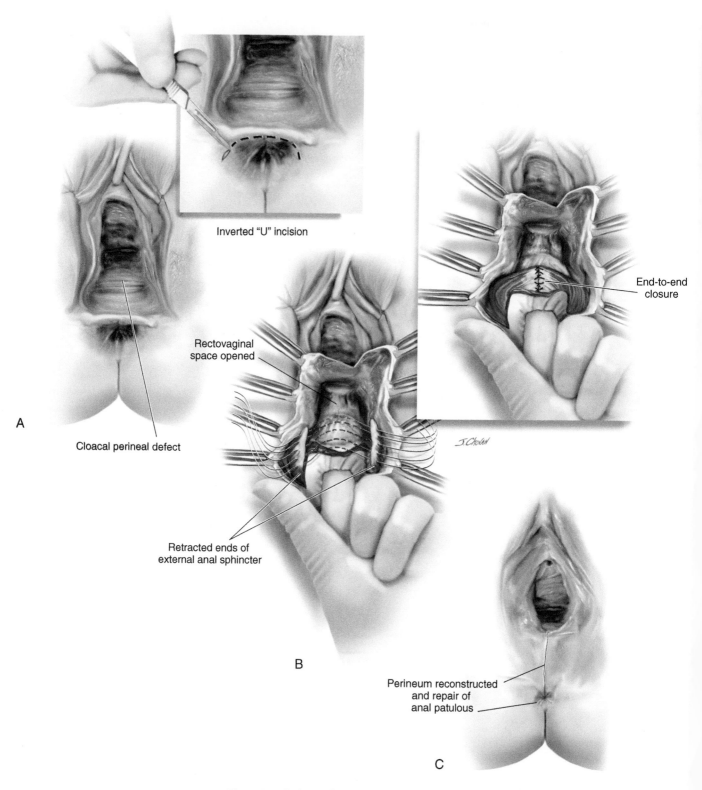

Inverted "U" incision

Cloacal perineal defect

A

Rectovaginal
space opened

Retracted ends of
external anal sphincter

B

End-to-end
closure

Perineum reconstructed
and repair of
anal patulous

C

Figure 9-11 Technique for end-to-end sphincteroplasty.

5. Frequently, a perineorrhaphy needs to be performed. In addition, if necessary, a rectocele and/or distal levatorplasty may be performed to decrease the size of the vaginal introitus. At the completion of the repair, the anal canal should be tightened to allow just an index finger to be admitted.

6. The skin edges are then closed with interrupted 3-0 absorbable sutures. The author of this text does not routinely place a drain in this area. Patients are maintained on stool softeners throughout the postoperative period.

Case 1: Repair of Symptomatic Rectocele

 View: Video 9-2

A 53-year-old patient has symptoms related to pelvic pressure with some tissue protrusion and difficulty evacuating her stools; she has to press on her perineum to evacuate her bowels fully. She underwent a hysterectomy for a benign gynecologic indication. She denies any lower urinary tract symptoms. She does, however, complain of some dyspareunia, which she relates to her prolapse symptoms. An examination confirms that she has good support of the anterior vaginal wall and vaginal cuff. A bulging of the posterior vaginal wall is revealed to the level of the hymen when she strains in a supine position. A thinning of the perineum and some perineal descent are also observed. Rectal examination confirms a rectocele, and the patient believes that the location of the examining finger is exactly where the stool gets trapped when she tries to evacuate her bowels. The patient desires surgical correction of the rectocele. Risks and benefits are discussed in great detail, and she understands that rectocele repair does not guarantee that her outlet obstructive symptoms will be completely resolved. She undergoes a rectocele repair with a perineoplasty. During the dissection of the anterior wall of the rectum off the posterior vaginal wall, an attempt is made to identify an enterocele sac; however, no peritoneal sac is identified and the apex is well supported. **(See Video 9-2, "Defect-Specific Rectocele Repair."**　)

Case Discussion

This patient's presentation is an example of a straightforward symptomatic rectocele that, in the author's opinion, did not require further evaluation. Her defecatory symptoms were typical of patients with a symptomatic rectocele and were easily reproduced with a clinical examination.

Case 2: Repair of Symptomatic Rectocele in Conjunction with Repair of Posterior Enterocele

 View: Video 9-3

A 48-year-old patient has a large posterior vaginal wall defect. She underwent a total abdominal hysterectomy (TAH) and a Burch colposuspension approximately 10 years before presentation. Her anterior vaginal wall is relatively foreshortened but well supported, as is her vaginal apex. She denies any significant bowel dysfunction and desires definitive therapy. A large prolapse of the entire posterior vaginal wall is revealed during examination, which is consistent with a posterior enterocele and a large rectocele. The plan is to proceed with a native tissue suture repair of this area, which will include an intraperitoneal vaginal vault suspension for the posterior enterocele, in the hopes of creating some extra vaginal length, as well as a defect-specific rectocele with an extensive perineoplasty. A vaginal dissection of the entire posterior vaginal wall is performed. An obvious enterocele is identified and entered, and uterosacral vaginal vault suspension is performed to suspend the uppermost portion of the posterior vaginal wall and to address the enterocele. The rectocele is corrected in a defect-specific fashion, followed by a distal levatorplasty and extensive perineoplasty. **(See Video 9-3, "Rectocele Repair in Conjunction with Repair of Posterior Enterocele."**　)

Case Discussion

Although this patient had no defecatory dysfunction, a large posterior vaginal prolapse existed. The patient obviously had the posterior vaginal prolapse in addition to the rectocele and enterocele; consequently, the authors of this text believed it is of great importance to dissect it out and treat it as one would treat any type of hernia by mobilizing and entering the peritoneal sac. An intraperitoneal suspension in such a case is ideal; in that the upper part of posterior vaginal wall can be resuspended to provide added length to the foreshortened anterior vaginal wall. A suspension to the sacrospinous ligament would have also been a reasonable option.

Case 3: Repair of Symptomatic Rectocele in Conjunction with Repair of Anal Sphincter

 View: Video 9-4

A 33-year-old patient complains of some stool evacuation difficulties, some pelvic pressure, and fecal incontinence. She relates all of these problems back to the delivery of her last child approximately 2 years before presentation. At that time, she had a third-degree tear that ultimately broke down and required a second repair. Her fecal incontinence is described as being somewhat infrequent; however, she routinely loses gas, and, if her stools are soft or of a liquid nature, she has difficulty controlling them. A thin perineum with a gaping introitus and an obvious rectocele are noted with examination. She has a good pelvic floor contraction on command. An endoluminal anal ultrasound is performed to evaluate her fecal incontinence further, which shows a defect in her anterior sphincter from approximately the 10- to the 2-o'clock position. Because she has good contraction of her pelvic floor muscle, no other physiologic testing in the form of pudendal nerve terminal motor latency studies or anal manometry is required.

A defect-specific rectocele repair and an end-to-end plication of the external and internal anal sphincter across the anterior surface of the rectum are performed. **(See Video 9-4, "Rectocele Repair in Conjunction with Repair of Anal Sphincter."** 🖐)

Case Discussion

Minimal testing was preoperatively performed to confirm the anal sphincter defect. Any testing related to the outlet obstruction was unnecessary; as the rectocele was symptomatic with prolapse-type symptoms and was going to be fixed at the time of the anal sphincter repair. Maintaining the patient on a soft diet for at least 2 weeks after the surgery is important. In addition, observing a little breakdown of the perineal incision after the sphincter repair is not uncommon as a result of the tenseness and pressure placed on the closure of the perineum. The type of sphincter procedure performed in this case was an end-to-end sphincteroplasty; as significant lateral retraction of the disrupted muscle ends was present.

Case 4: Rectocele and Enterocele Repair Augmented with Biologic Mesh

 View: Video 9-5

A 53-year-old patient has recurrent pelvic organ prolapse after a vaginal hysterectomy; an anterior and posterior repair was performed approximately 6 months before presentation. Her prolapse is secondary to a defect in the posterior vaginal wall. She also complains of some stool trapping, as well as significant dyspareunia, which seems to be mostly introital dyspareunia. A high rectocele with possibly an enterocele, a somewhat foreshortened vagina, and a vaginal constriction ring are noted during examination. After a detailed discussion with the patient, it was decided to proceed with a suture repair of the posterior vaginal prolapse. To prevent the formation of any further vaginal constriction, a biologic graft (Surgisis Biodesign) was used to bridge the defects in need of support and possibly to replace the vaginal epithelium, if necessary. Enterocele repair with a vaginal vault suspension and augmentation of the upper part of the posterior vaginal wall are performed to address the high rectocele without creating any vaginal constriction. Distal rectocele repair and perineoplasty were also performed. **(See Video 9-5, "Rectocele and Enterocele Repair Augmented with Biologic Mesh."** 🎥**)**

Case Discussion

This patient had numerous functional and anatomic complaints. The functional complaints were related to sexual dysfunction from the constriction band, as well as outlet obstruction symptoms secondary to a recurrent rectocele. Because the prolapse symptoms were going to be corrected, regardless of what would be shown on any imaging studies, the author decided to proceed with correcting the anatomy; if residual defecation symptoms persisted, then they would be evaluated.

Case 5: Symptomatic Rectocele in Conjuction with a Large Sigmoidocele

A 68-year-old woman complains of difficulty evacuating stool and splinting with bowel movements, as well as a feeling of fullness in her vagina. She recently examined her genitalia with a mirror and described a golf ball–sized protrusion on straining. She denies any urinary symptoms but recently had a urinary tract infection for which she was successfully treated. After a physical examination, it is determined that the patient has a stage I cystocele and urethral hypermobility with straining at an angle of 50 degrees with the use of the cotton-tipped swab (Q-tip) test. Her uterus is well supported, but she also has a stage III rectocele and perineal thinning. The large rectocele is clearly appreciated during a rectal examination. She denies any rectal or vaginal bleeding; however, she is guaiac positive. A multichannel cystometrogram shows normal filling capacity with a stable detrusor and a normal voiding curve. She has a small amount of stress incontinence with prolapse reduction. Although the patient desires to have the rectocele fixed, it is believed that she should be evaluated for the guaiac-positive stool before performing any surgical intervention. Colonoscopy and defecography are performed, which notes a large sigmoidocele with the question of intussusception of the sigmoid into the upper rectum (Figure 9-12).

After consultation with a colorectal surgical specialist, surgical options are discussed. Plans to proceed with posterior repair, perineoplasty, and the transobturator tape (TOT) procedure are made, in conjunction with a sigmoid resection performed by colorectal surgery. The patient tolerates the procedure well and is discharged on postoperative day 3. She has complete resolution of her defecatory dysfunction in that she no longer has to splint to evacuate her stools.

Case Discussion

This case clearly demonstrated the importance of a multidisciplinary approach to the pelvic floor. If the patient would not have had a colorectal evaluation, her symptoms would most likely have persisted, secondary to the lack of attention to the sigmoidocele.

Outcomes of Posterior Vaginal Wall Repair

Midline Plication or Traditional Posterior Colporrhaphy

The reported anatomic success rates with this type of repair range from 76% to 96% with *de novo* development of dyspareunia ranging from 4% to 26% (Table 9-1).

Site-Specific Defect Repair

This technique is similar to the traditional posterior repair in terms of dissection. The goal of the repair is for the surgeon to identify and individually correct breaks in the rectovaginal septum. Tradition levatorplasty is avoided. Anatomic cure with this procedure ranges from 56% to 100% (Table 9-2).

Paraiso and colleagues (2006) compared three techniques for rectocele repair in a prospective randomized trial. Patients were randomized to receive a traditional repair

Figure 9-12 Intussusception requires an evaluation by a colorectal specialist, as well as by other appropriate subspecialists, if associated with multiple pelvic floor complaints. As depicted, the rectal mucosa may slip within itself, creating a fold that narrows the canal.

(From Hull TL: Posterior pelvic floor abnormalities. In Karram M, editor: Atlas of pelvic anatomy and gynecologic surgery *Philadelphia, 2011, Elsevier.)*

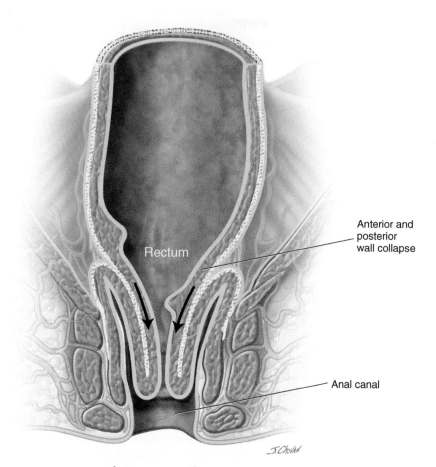

Rectum

Anterior and posterior wall collapse

Anal canal

J.Chovan

Intussusception

($n = 37$), a site-specific repair ($n = 37$), or a site-specific repair augmented with porcine small intestine mucosa ($n = 32$). All patients preoperatively had stage II or greater posterior vaginal wall prolapse. The objective anatomic failure rate was highest in the graft-augmented group (12 to 26) at 1 year after surgery, which was statistically significantly worse than the results in the site-specific group (6 of 27) and in the traditional repair group (4 of 28). No significant differences in subjective symptoms (worsening prolapse or colorectal symptoms) or dyspareunia were revealed among the three groups.

Transanal Repair of Rectocele

Three trials have evaluated transanal versus transvaginal repairs of rectoceles. (Kahn et al, 1999; Nieminen et al, 2004; Farid, 2010) Each trial had slightly different inclusion criteria. Kahn included women who had symptoms of prolapse or impaired rectal evacuation with incomplete emptying on isotope defecography and normal compliance on anorectal manometry. The Nieminen study included women with symptomatic rectoceles not responding to conservative therapy. Importantly, women with compromised anal sphincter function and other symptomatic genital prolapse were excluded. In both trials the vaginal repair was performed by gynecologists and the transanal repair by colorectal surgeons. In the Kahn trial, the posterior vaginal wall repair was performed using levator plication; in the Nieminen trial, the rectovaginal fascia was plicated. Farid's inclusion criteria required women to have a rectocele larger than 2 cm

Table 9-1 Outcomes of Studies Looking at Midline Plication Repair of Rectocele

Study (year)	N	Mean Follow-Up (months)	Anatomic Cure (%)	Vaginal Bulge (%)	Vaginal Digitation (%)	Defecatory Dysfunction (%)	Dyspareunia (%)
Arnold, 1990							
Preoperative	29				20		
Postoperative	24		80			36	23
Mellgren et al, 1995							
Preoperative	25			21	50	8	
Postoperative	25	12	96	4	0	8	8
Kahn and Stanton, 1997							
Preoperative	231			64		4	
Postoperative	171	42	76	31	33	11	16
Weber, 2000							
Preoperative	53	12					
Postoperative	53						26
Sand et al, 2001							
Preoperative	70	12					
Postoperative	67		90				
Maher et al, 2004							
Preoperative	38			100	100	3	37
Postoperative	38	12	87	5	16	0	5
Abramov et al, 2005							
Preoperative	183			100		17	8
Postoperative	183	>12	82	4		18	17
Paraiso et al, 2006							
Preoperative	37	17.5	86			80	56
Postoperative	28					32	45

Table 9-2 Outcome of Studies Looking at Site-Specific Defect Repair of Rectocele

Study (year)	N	Mean Follow-Up (months)	Anatomic Cure (%)	Vaginal Bulge (%)	Vaginal Digitation (%)	Defecatory Dysfunction (%)	Dyspareunia (%)
Cundiff et al, 1998							
Preoperative	69	12		100	39	13	29
Postoperative	61		82	81	18	8	19
Porter et al, 1999							
Preoperative	125	6		38	24	24	67
Postoperative	72		82	14	21	21	46
Kenton, 1999							
Preoperative	66	12		86	30	30	28
Postoperative	46		90	9	15		8
Glavind and Madsen, 2000							
Preoperative	67	3					12
Postoperative	67		100				3
Singh, 2003							
Preoperative	42	18		78		9	31
Postoperative	33		92	7		5	15
Abramov et al, 2005							
Preoperative	124			100		15	8
Postoperative	124	>12	56	11		19	16
Paraiso et al, 2006							
Preoperative	37	17.5	78		58		48
Postoperative	27				21		28

on defecography with symptoms including digitation, incomplete evacuation, excessive straining, and dyspareunia. Women with a compromised anal sphincter complex or recurrent prolapse, rectal prolapse, intussusception, or anismus were excluded. The surgery was performed within the surgical department, and blinded examiners used defecography, anal manometry, and a modified obstructed defecation syndrome questionnaire to report outcomes.

On the basis of these three trials, the results for transvaginal repair of the rectocele are superior to transanal rectocele repair in terms of subjective and objective outcomes. In women with rectocele alone, recurrent rectocele occurred in 2 out of 39 women in the vaginal group and in 7 out of 48 after the transanal repair, a difference that did not reach statistical significance. Postoperative enterocele was, however, significantly less common after vaginal surgery, as compared with the transanal group.

Farid and colleagues (2010) reported on the outcomes of the three types of rectocele repair, comparing transperineal repair with levatorplasty and transanal repair and noted conclusions similar to the two previously discussed trials. The size of the rectocele on defecographic examination was significantly smaller in the transperineal group (with or without levatorplasty), as compared with the transanal repair. In addition, the functional outcome, based on a modified obstruction defecation syndrome questionnaire, was better after transperineal repair as compared with transanal repair.

Thornton and associates (2005) reported in a single nonrandomized study outcomes for a cohort of women with symptomatic rectocele who were treated laparoscopically ($n = 40$) versus transanally ($n = 40$). Level 2B evidence from this study supports the superiority of the transanal approach for symptomatic relief (55% versus 28%, $p <0.02$) but lower postoperative dyspareunia rates (22% versus 36%) with the laparoscopic approach.

van Dam and colleagues (2000) reported a combined transvaginal and transanal repair in 89 women who were evaluated at a follow-up of 52 months. The anatomic success rate was 71% (defined as no persistent or recurrent rectocele on defecography at 6 months). However, *de novo* dyspareunia was reported in 41% of women, and a deterioration of fecal maintenance was reported in seven patients.

Mesh-Augmented Rectocele

Sand and associates (2001) compared posterior repair with and without mesh and noted rectocele recurrence appeared equally with and without polyglactin (Vicryl) mesh augmentation (7 out of 67 versus 6 out of 65). Paraiso and colleagues (2006) also noted no benefit to augmenting a site-specific repair with a porcine small intestine graft overlay. Neither trial reported any mesh erosion.

Recently, Sung and associates (2012) reported a double-blinded multicenter randomized control trial comparing native tissue repair or native tissue repair augmented with porcine subintestinal submucosal (SIS) graft overlay for symptomatic grade 2 rectocele. The native tissue repair involved either a midline plication or a site-specific repair. No differences among the groups were observed in the objective and subjective success rates or in the resolution of defecatory symptoms at one year follow-up. Postoperative dyspareunia rates were not significantly different (7% in the native tissue group versus 12.5% in the graft group).

Modified Sacrocolpopexy

The abdominal route is used in the correction of posterior vaginal wall prolapse when a co-existing apical defect requires surgery. The technique is a modification of sacrocolpopexy with an extension of the posterior mesh down to the distal posterior vaginal wall and/or the perineal body. The procedure has been reported completely abdominally or as a combined abdominal and vaginal approach. Table 9-3 summarizes a series of studies that have reported on extended posterior fixation of sacrocolpopexy mesh.

Table 9-3 Abdominal Repair (Posterior Extension of Colpopexy Mesh)

				Dyspareunia	
Author	Number	Follow-Up (in months)	Success	Preoperative	Postoperative
Baessler, 2001	33	26	45%	39%	13%
Fox, 2000	29	14	90%	38%	17%
Su, 2007	122	12	90%	—	—
Lyons, 1997	20	12	80%	—	—
Marinkovic, 2003	12	39	91%	29%	none

SUMMARY:

- Transvaginal repair of a rectocele continues to be reported as either a traditional repair or site-specific repair without a good anatomic basis for the descriptive nature of these procedures. Similar anatomic outcomes are reported with both types of repairs with a trend toward a higher dyspareunia rate when levatorplasty is used.
- A transvaginal approach appears to be superior to the transanal approach for the repair of a rectocele.
- Minimal data exist for outcomes related to the repair of an enterocele either alone or in conjunction with a rectocele repair.
- To date, no study has shown any benefit to mesh overlay or augmentation of a suture repair for posterior vaginal wall prolapse.
- Although modified abdominal sacrocolpopexy results have been reported, data are lacking on how these results would compare with the traditional transvaginal repair of posterior vaginal wall prolapse.

Suggested Readings

Abramov Y, Gandhi S, Goldberg RP, et al: Site-specific rectocele repair compared with standard posterior colporrhaphy, *Obstet Gynecol* 105(2):314–318, 2005.

Arnold MW, Stewart WR, Aguilar PS: Rectocele repair. Four years' experience, *Dis Colon Rectum* 33(8):684–687, 1990.

Baessler K, Schuessler B: Abdominal sacrocolpopexy and anatomy and function of the posterior compartment, *Obstet Gynecol* 97(5 Pt 1):678–684, 2001.

Boyles SH, Weber AM, Meyn L: Procedures for pelvic organ prolapse in the United States, 1979-1997, *Am J Obstet Gynecol* 108–115, 2003.

Burrows LJ, Meyn LA, Walters MD, et al: Pelvic symptoms in women with pelvic organ prolapse, *Obstet Gynecol* 104:982–988, 2004.

Cundiff GW, Weidner AC, Visco AG, et al: An anatomic and functional assessment of the discrete defect rectocele repair, *Am J Obstet Gynecol* 179(6 Pt 1):1451–1456; discussion 1456-1457, 1998.

DeLancey JO: Structural anatomy of the posterior pelvic compartment as it relates to rectocele, *Am J Obstet Gynecol* 180:815–823, 1999.

Ellerkmann RM, Cundiff GW, Melick CF, et al: Correlation of symptoms with location and severity of pelvic organ prolapse, *Am J Obstet Gynecol* 185:1332–1337, 2001.

Farid M, Madbouly KM, Hussein A, et al: Randomized controlled trial between perineal and anal repairs of rectocele in obstructed defecation, *World J Surg* 34:822–829, 2010.

Farrell SA, Dempsey T, Geldenhuys L: Histologic examination of "fascia" used in colporrhaphy, *Obstet Gynecol* 98:794–798, 2001

Fenner DE: Diagnosis and assessment of sigmoidoceles, *Am J Obstet Gynecol* 175:1438–1441; discussion 1441–1442, 1996.

Fox SD, Stanton SL: Vault prolapse and rectocele: assessment of repair using sacrocolpopexy with mesh interposition, *BJOG* 107(11):1371–1375, 2000.

Francis WJ, Jeffcoate TN: Dyspareunia following vaginal operations, *J Obstet Gynaecol Br Commonw* 68:1–10, 1961.

Glavind K, Madsen H: A prospective study of the discrete fascial defect rectocele repair, *Acta Obstet Gynecol Scand* 79:145–147, 2000.

Jeffcoate TN: Posterior colpoperineorrhaphy, *Am J Obstet Gynecol* 77:490–502, 1959.

Kahn MA, Stanton SL: Posterior colporrhaphy: its effects on bowel and sexual function, *BJOG* 104:82–86, 1997.

Kahn MA, Stanton SL, Kumar D, et al: Posterior colporrhaphy is superior to the transanal repair for the treatment of posterior vaginal wall prolapse, *Neurourol Urodyn* 18(4):329–330, 1999.

Kenton K, Shott S, Brubaker L: Outcome after rectovaginal fascia reattachment for rectocele repair, *Am J Obstet Gynecol* 181(6):1360–1363, 1999.

Lewicky-Gaupp C, Fenner DE, DeLancey JOL: Posterior vaginal wall repair: Does anatomy matter? *Contemporary OB/GYN* 54(10):44–49, 2009.

Lyons TL, Winer WK: Laparoscopic rectocele repair using polyglactin mesh, *J Am Assoc Gynecol Laparosc* 4(3):381–384, 1997.

Maher C, Qatawneh AM, Baessler K, et al: Midline rectovaginal fascial plication for repair of rectocele and obstructed defecation, *Obstet Gynecol* 104(4):685–689, 2004.

Marinkovic SP, Stanton SL: Triple compartment prolapse: sacrocolpopexy with anterior and posterior mesh extensions, *BJOG* 110(3):323–326, 2003.

Mellgren A, Anzén B, Nilsson BY, et al: Results of rectocele repair. A prospective study, *Dis Colon Rectum* 38(1):7–13, 1995.

Nieminen K, Hiltunen KM, Laitinen J, et al: Transanal or vaginal approach to rectocele repair: a prospective, randomized pilot study, *Dis Colon Rectum* 47(10):1636–1642, 2004.

Paraiso MF, Barber MD, Muir TW, et al: Rectocele repair: a randomized trial of three surgical techniques including graft augmentation, *Am J Obstet Gynecol* 195(6):1762–1771, 2006.

Porter WE, Steele A, Walsh P, et al: The anatomic and functional outcomes of defect-specific rectocele repairs, *Am J Obstet Gynecol* 181(6):1353–1358, 1999.

Puigdollers A, Fernández-Fraga X, Azpiroz F: persistent symptoms of functional outlet obstruction after rectocele repair, *Colorectal Dis* 9(3):262–265, 2007.

Richardson AC: The rectovaginal septum revisited; its relationship to rectocele and its importance in rectocele repair, *Clin Obstet Gynaecol* 36:976–983, 1993.

Sand PK, Koduri S, Lobel RW, et al: Prospective randomized trial of polyglactin 910 mesh to prevent recurrence of cystoceles and rectoceles, *Am J Obstet Gynecol* 184:1357–1362, 2001.

Silva WA, Pauls RN, Segal JL, et al: Uterosacral ligament vault suspension; five year outcomes, *Obstet Gynecol* 108:255–263, 2006.

Singh K, Cortes E, Reid WM: Evaluation of the fascial technique for surgical repair of isolated posterior vaginal wall prolapse, *Obstet Gynecol* 101(2):320–324, 2003.

Su KC, Mutone MF, Terry CL, et al: Abdominovaginal sacral colpoperineopexy; patient perceptions, anatomical outcomes, and graft erosions, *Int Urogynecol J Pelvic Floor Dysfunct* 18:503–511, 2007.

Sung VW, Rardin CR, Raker CA, et al: Porcine subintestinal submucosal graft augmentation for rectocele repair: a randomized controlled trial, *Obstet Gynecol* 119(1):125–133, 2012.

Thornton MJ, Lam A, King DW: Laparoscopic or transanal repair of rectocele? A retrospective matched cohort study, *Dis Colon Rectum* 48:792–798, 2005.

van Dam JH, Huisman WM, Hop WC, et al: Fecal continence after rectocele repair: a prospective study, *Int J Colorectal Dis* 15(1):54–57, 2000.

Weber AM, Walters MD, Piedmonte MR: Sexual function and vaginal anatomy in women before and after surgery for pelvic organ prolapse and urinary incontinence, *Am J Obstet Gynecol* 182:1610–1615, 2000.

Obliterative Procedures for Pelvic Organ Prolapse

10

Janelle Evans MD and Mickey Karram MD

 Video Clips online

10-1 Le Fort Partial Colpocleisis
10-2 Complete Colpectomy and Colpocleisis (Example 1)

10-3 Complete Colpectomy and Colpocleisis (Example 2)

As women live longer and healthier lives, pelvic floor disorders are becoming prevalent and increasingly important health and social issues. An estimated 63 million women will be 45 years old or older by 2030, and 33% of the population will be postmenopausal by 2050. In the United States, the largest segment of the population growth-wise is the woman above 60 years of age. Approximately 10% of women will undergo surgery at some point for pelvic organ prolapse or incontinence. Some studies have noted a reoperation rate for failures up to 30%, mainly in the anterior compartment. As a result of an increasing number of women entering the eighth and ninth decades of life, these individuals often develop symptomatic pelvic organ prolapse often after unsuccessful attempts at pessary therapy or surgery. These women frequently have concomitant medical issues and are not sexually active, making extensive surgery less than ideal. Procedures have been described to alleviate the symptoms of pelvic organ prolapse by obliterating the vaginal canal. Specifically, these procedures are classified as a Le Fort partial colpocleisis, in which the patient maintains her uterus in place, and a partial or complete colpectomy and colpocleisis is performed in the patient after hysterectomy. This chapter discusses the indications and techniques of these procedures.

Le Fort Partial Colpocleisis

A Le Fort partial colpocleisis is an option if the patient has her uterus and is no longer sexually active. Because the uterus is retained, evaluating any future uterine bleeding or cervical pathologic abnormalities is difficult. Therefore endovaginal ultrasound, endometrial biopsy, and Papanicolaou smear (Pap smear) must be performed before surgery. (Denehy et al, 1995) The ideal candidate for such a procedure is the patient who has complete uterine procidentia with symmetric eversion of the anterior and posterior vaginal walls (Figure 10-1).

Case 1: Le Fort Partial Colpocleisis

 View: Video 10-1

An 82-year-old woman has symptomatic pelvic organ prolapse, secondary to a protrusion of her uterus and eversion of the vagina well beyond the introitus. Her medical history is complicated by

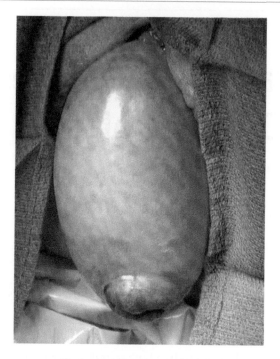

Figure 10-1 Complete procidentia.

chronic obstructive pulmonary disease and hypertension. She is widowed and has no interest in becoming sexually active in the future. After two previous attempts at pessary therapy, which failed secondary to her inability to maintain the pessary in place, she seeks definitive therapy. Her pelvic examination notes a complete uterine procidentia with the cervix extending 8 centimeters beyond the introitus and symmetric eversion of the anterior and posterior vaginal walls. She also complains of some recent voiding dysfunction and difficulty emptying her bladder. A simple office filling study documents a void of 200 ml with a residual of 120 ml. She is then filled to a maximum capacity of 250 ml; the sign of stress incontinence is not shown with or without a reduction of the prolapse. She has had a recent negative Pap smear, and an endometrial biopsy in the office notes an atrophic endometrium. After a detailed discussion, plans are made to proceed with a Le Fort partial colpocleisis, a Kelly-Kennedy plication of the bladder neck, and a levatorplasty and perineoplasty. Because of her chronic obstructive pulmonary disease, this procedure is to be performed under monitored anesthesia care (MAC) anesthesia with a pudendal block placed and local infiltration of an anesthetic.

Procedural Steps

1. The procedure is begun by placing the cervix on traction to evert the vagina. The vaginal mucosa is injected with 0.025% bupivacaine or 2% Lidocaine with 1:200,000 epinephrine just below the vaginal epithelium. A Foley catheter with a 5- to 10-ml balloon is placed in the bladder for identification of the bladder neck.

2. The areas that are to be denuded are marked anteriorly and posteriorly. The area should extend from approximately 2 cm from the tip of the cervix to 4 to 5 cm below the external urethral meatus. A mirror image on the posterior aspect of the cervix and vagina are also identified.

3. The previously outlined areas are removed by sharp dissection (Figure 10-2, *A* and *C*). The surgeon should leave the maximum amount of muscularis behind on the bladder and rectum. Hemostasis is an absolute must. While removing the posterior vaginal flap, one should not attempt to enter the peritoneum. If the peritoneum is inadvertently entered, the defect should be closed with an interrupted delayed absorbable suture.

4. The cut edges of the anterior and posterior vaginal walls are sewn together with interrupted delayed absorbable sutures. The knot should be turned into the epithelium-lined tunnels, when possible, which have been created bilaterally (see Figure 10-2, *D-E*). After the vagina has

been inverted, superior and inferior margins of the rectangle can be sutured together (see Figure 10-2, *F*).

5. In the author's opinion, a plication of the bladder neck or a synthetic midurethral sling should be routinely performed because of the high incidence of postoperative stress incontinence (see Figure 10-2, *B*). (Denehy et al, 1995) In addition, an aggressive perineorrhaphy with a distal levator plication should be performed to narrow the introitus, decrease the caliber of the genital hiatus, and build up the perineum. For the technique of levatorplasty, see page 172. (**See Video 10-1, "Le Fort Partial Colpocleisis,"** for a video demonstration of the procedure.)

Case Discussion

In general, approximately 90% to 95% of patients will have complete relief of symptoms with good anatomic results after undergoing a Le Fort partial colpocleisis. Complete breakdown or partial recurrence can be expected in 2% to 5% of patients, which is mostly because of either poor hemostasis with hematoma formation or an infectious process. Goldman and colleagues (1985)

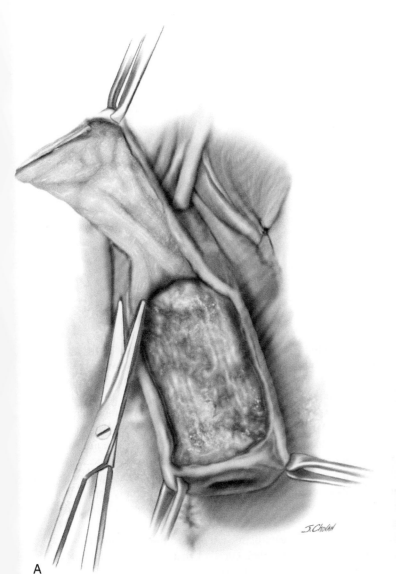

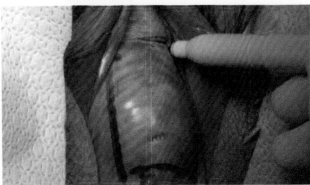

A

Figure 10-2 A, Denuding of the anterior vaginal epithelium.

Continued

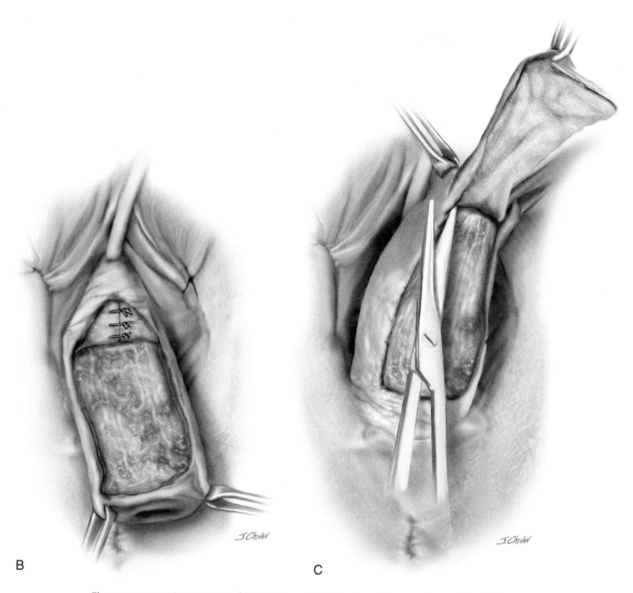

B

C

Figure 10-2, cont'd. B, Plication of the bladder neck. **C,** Denuding of the posterior vaginal epithelium.

reported results and complications from a modified Le Fort partial colpocleisis in 118 patients; 91% of the patients had good anatomic results, whereas 85% had complete relief of symptoms, 2.5% had recurrence of their prolapse, 10.2% developed incontinence or a worsening of their incontinence, and 1.8% had late vaginal bleeding.

In general, postoperative complications are low in comparison with vaginal hysterectomy and compartmental repairs. *De novo* stress urinary incontinence is a known risk after obliterative procedures and should be thoroughly evaluated preoperatively with urodynamic testing to ensure that the patient has a normal postvoid residual volume and no evidence of genuine or occult incontinence. (Fitzgerald, 2003) Both the surgeon and the subspecialists should thoroughly assess the postoperative risks of thromboembolic events, cardiovascular issues, and other systemic abnormalities in the patient with multiple co-morbidities to ensure an appropriate surgical and anesthesia plan. (Gerten et al, 2008)

In the opinion of the authors, a concomitant levatorplasty and perineorrhaphy should be a component of any Le Fort colpocleisis because of the theoretical risk that anatomic failure may be minimized by supporting the perineum with a tighter pelvic outlet as well as decreasing the size of the genital hiatus.

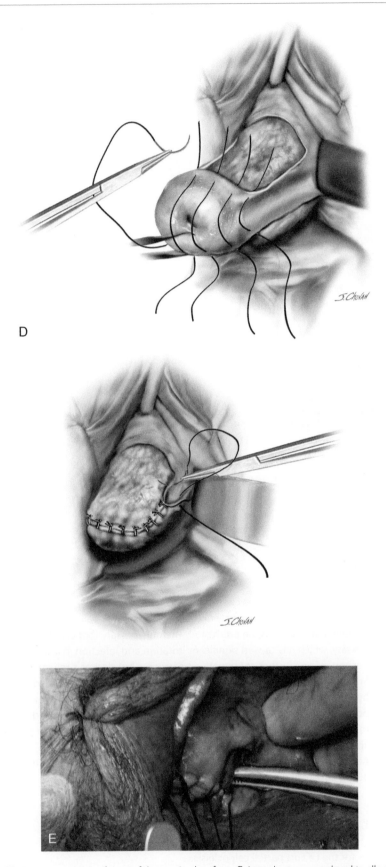

Figure 10-2, cont'd. D, Approximation of most of the proximal surfaces. **E,** Lateral sutures are placed to allow for drainage canals.

Continued

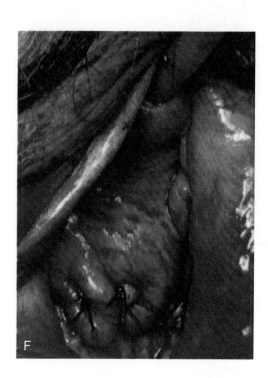

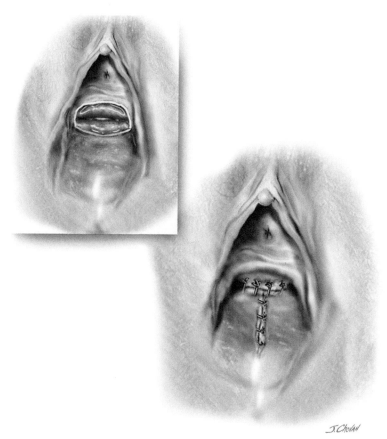

Figure 10-2, cont'd. F, Distal sutures are placed to complete the colpocleisis.

(Drawings modified from Baggish MS, Karram MM: Atlas of pelvic anatomy and gynecologic surgery, *ed 3, St Louis, 2011, Elsevier.)*

Case 2: Complete Colpectomy and Colpocleisis

 View: Video 10-2

An 89-year-old woman has posthysterectomy vault prolapse involving a large cystocele and rectocele. She is symptomatic with the prolapse and has significant defecatory and urinary tract dysfunction related to the protrusion. The only pessary that can be maintained is a large donut pessary, which has caused significant irritation and infection in a short period. The patient is not desirous of any further conservative treatments but desires a minimally invasive surgical approach. She does not intend to be sexually active and has no significant medical issues except chronic hypertension, which is well controlled with medication. A physical examination confirms a large posthysterectomy prolapse that descends approximately 8 cm outside the introitus. The vaginal mucosa is atrophic. Lower urinary tract evaluation notes an elevated postvoid residual volume of approximately 150 ml. No occult incontinence is demonstrated with a reduction of the prolapse. Additionally, she has significant stool in the lower portion of the rectum, which is consistent with outlet obstruction from her large rectocele.

Procedural Steps

1. The most prominent portion of the prolapse is grasped with two Allis clamps. The vaginal epithelium is injected with a 1% Lidocaine with epinephrine solution as previously mentioned for the Le Fort partial colpocleisis.

2. The vagina is circumscribed by an incision several centimeters from the hymen at the base of the prolapse. A marking pencil is then used to mark rectangular portions of the vagina that will be removed sharply. The vaginal epithelium is completely removed. An effort is made to avoid entering the peritoneal cavity (Figure 10-3, *A-B*).

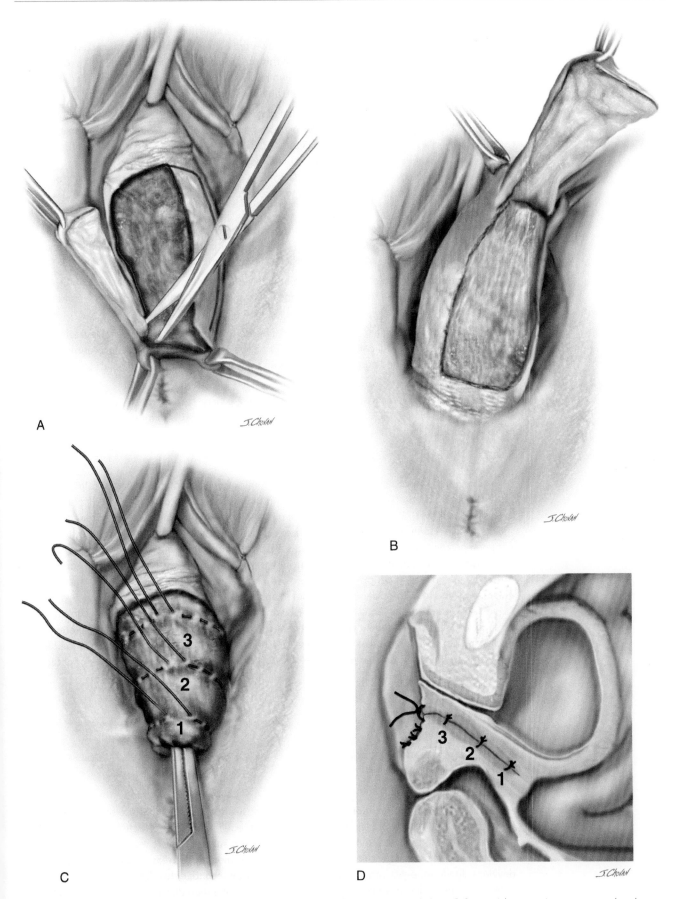

Figure 10-3 A, Denuding of the anterior vaginal epithelium. **B,** Denuding of the posterior epithelium. **C,** Sequential purse-string sutures are placed.
D, Colpocleisis procedure is completed.

(Modified from Baggish MS, Karram MM: Atlas of pelvic anatomy and gynecologic surgery, ed 3. St Louis, 2011, Elsevier.)

3. A series of purse-string sutures are placed, sequentially inverting the vagina by tying the sutures (Figure 10-3, *C*). The apex of the soft tissue is inverted by the tip of a forceps as each purse-string suture is tied (Figure 10-3, *D*). A variation of this procedure can involve performing a separate anterior and posterior colporrhaphy with two purse-string sutures to close the anterior and posterior segments together and obliterate any dead space between compartments.

4. Levatorplasty is then performed; the genital hiatus is invariably widened in this patient population. The puborectalis and pubococcygeus muscles are reapproximated in the midline with delayed absorbable sutures (see Figures 10-3, *A-D*), creating a shelf above the rectum as a theoretical barrier to visceral descent. (For technique depiction, the reader is referred to page 172.) **(See Videos 10-2 and 10-3, "Complete Colpectomy and Colpocleisis,"** for demonstrations of total colpectomy and total colpocleisis with levatorplasty.

Technique of Distal Levatorplasty with High Colpoperineorrhaphy

1. Two Allis clamps are placed superiorly on the genital hiatus to demarcate the lateral edges of the extent of tissue removal from the posterior fourchette (Figure 10-4, *A*).

2. A diamond-shaped flap of epithelium is marked over the distal posterior vaginal wall proximally and perineal skin distally. The marked perineal skin and vaginal epithelium is sharply removed (see Figure 10-4, *A*)

3. The distal posterior vaginal wall is mobilized laterally to allow access to the distal levator and muscle. Two to three 0-Vicryl sutures on a CT-1 needle are used to plicate the levator muscles across the midline, thus significantly decreasing the caliber of the distal vaginal canal (Figure 10-4, *A (inset), B-C*).

4. The perineal body is reconstructed using a series of 2-0 Vicryl sutures, greatly reducing the size of the genital hiatus. The vaginal and perineal skin is then closed with interrupted or running 3-0 Vicryl sutures (Figure 10-4, *D*).

Case Discussion

In general, total colpectomy and colpocleisis has a similar outcome to Le Fort partial colpocleisis with complications often related to patient comorbidities. Stepp and colleagues (2005) found that among women over 75 years of age with prolapse who underwent a full range of surgeries including colpectomy, most complications were related to medical comorbidities. The most common postoperative medical complications are pulmonary edema and congestive heart failure. Preoperative risk factors for complications include the length of surgery and a history of coronary artery disease, as well as peripheral vascular disease. DeLancey and Morely (1997) performed colpectomy and total colpocleisis on 33 women and reported a worsening of congestive heart failure in 2 women, urinary tract infection in 2 women, and pneumonia in 1 woman. Recurrent prolapse developed in 1 patient requiring repeat colpocleisis. A small risk (0% to 2%) of ureteric occlusion or injury may exist with obliterative procedures, usually as a result of kinking in the distal ureter. Almost all of these cases will resolve with the removal of the purse-string suture or plication stitch.

Case 3: Complete Colpectomy and Colpocleisis after Two Previous Attempts at Colpocleisis

 View: Video 10-3

A 79-year-old patient has recurrent pelvic organ prolapse after two prior colpocleises. The patient has a complicated history of invasive vulvar carcinoma requiring radical vulvectomy in which the majority of the urethra was removed. This procedure has resulted in severe incontinence, and an ileal conduit diversion of her urinary tract has been performed for this reason. She subsequently develops significant pelvic organ prolapse, which is mostly secondary to a large recurrent enterocele, and undergoes a colpectomy and colpocleisis. She then developed a second recurrent enterocele and again underwent repeat colpectomy and colpocleisis. On examination, she is noted to have an extremely thin vaginal epithelium behind which small bowel could be palpated. After a detailed discussion with the patient, she consents for attempt at a third colpectomy and colpocleisis with the understanding that the peritoneum will need to be entered to reduce the small bowel. A thorough discussion regarding the risk of small bowel injury is conducted before consent.Surgical Procedure

1. The initial steps taken are identical to those previously described for colpectomy and colpocleisis.

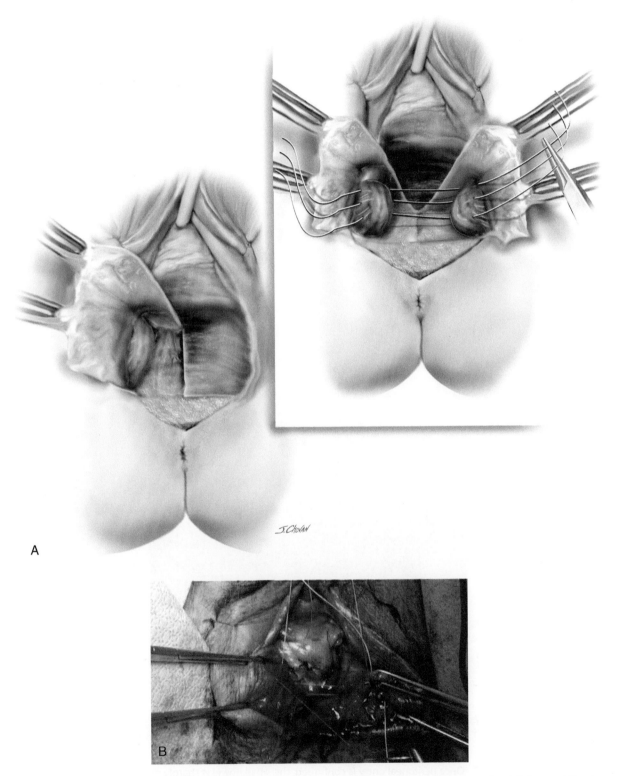

Figure 10-4 A, Lateral dissection to the levator ani muscles. Levator ani muscles are plicated with sequential sutures *(inset)*. **B,** Sequential levator plication sutures are placed.

Continued

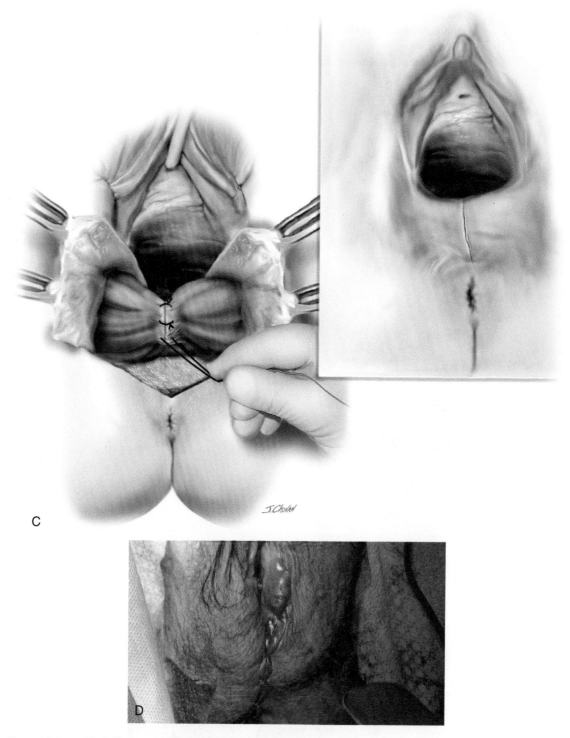

Figure 10-4, cont'd. C, Plication sutures are secured. Complete levatorplasty is demonstrated *(inset).* **D,** Colpocleisis and levatorplasty are completed.

(Parts A and C: Modified from Baggish MS, Karram MM: Atlas of pelvic anatomy and gynecologic surgery, ed 3, St Louis, 2011, Elsevier.)

2. Once the entire vaginal epithelium is removed, a finger is placed in the rectum and the enterocele sac is dissected away from the anterior vaginal wall and rectum to enter the peritoneum.

3. Once peritoneal entry is confirmed, the small bowel is sharply dissected off the peritoneum and reduced up into the pelvis.

4. Numerous purse-string sutures are then used to close down the enterocele sac. These sutures involve taking wide bites through the remnants of the uterosacral cardinal ligament complex to obliterate the neck of the enterocele completely.

5. The vaginal incision is closed with interrupted delayed absorbable sutures, and a distal levatorplasty and perineoplasty is performed as previously described (see Figure 10-4, *A-D*).

Case Discussion

This patient had multiple recurrences of her vaginal prolapse as a result of a lack of aggressively reducing and supporting an apical enterocele, which is a common result caused by the failure to plicate the levator muscles for support after removing the vaginal mucosa. An aggressive levatorplasty with complete obliteration of the central and distal vagina may have prevented these recurrences.

Quality of Life and Regret of Loss of Sexual Function

Barber and others (2006) found that obliterative procedures for stage III or IV pelvic organ prolapse significantly improved the quality of life as measured by several standardized questionnaires. Preoperative counseling should involve the discussion of the sexual implications of vaginal obliteration. Harmanli and associates (2003) reported no postoperative cases of regret after 41 consecutive cases of total colpocleisis. However, von Pechmann and colleagues (2003) reported regret over the loss of coital ability in eight women (12.9%). However, four of the eight stated that they still would have had the procedure if asked again.

Agarwala and colleagues (2007) described a 95% satisfaction rate after obliterative prolapse repairs in which all patients underwent a concomitant tension-free vaginal tape (TVT) procedure. The majority of the patients had improved stress urinary incontinence, and no postoperative voiding dysfunction was reported. In another study comparing satisfaction outcomes after obliterative prolapse repairs with traditional reconstructive procedures, there were similar overall postoperative scores in standardized surgeries as measured by validated questionnaires such as Urogenital Distress Inventory (UDI)–6 and Incontinence Impact Questionnaire (IIQ)–7. (Murphy, 2008)

Urinary Function after Obliterative Procedures

The challenge of the pelvic surgeon is to provide effective treatment for pelvic organ prolapse while maintaining and restoring lower urinary tract function. *De novo* stress incontinence is a recognized potential outcome of obliterative procedures. The risk of worsening any preexisting urinary retention with an antiincontinence procedure must be weighed against the risk of postcolpocleisis stress incontinence if an antiincontinence procedure is not performed. Surprisingly, many older women with advanced prolapse have normal urinary tract function but are at high risk for postoperative irritative symptoms and retention if a suburethral sling is performed.

Fitzgerald and Brubaker (2003) retrospectively reviewed the results of colpocleisis with particular attention to perioperative stress incontinence. They demonstrated a 36% incidence of elevated postvoid residual volumes (>100 ml) in 64 patients. Preoperatively, stress incontinence was diagnosed in 78% of those tested, and an occult incontinence was diagnosed in 33%. The majority of studies does not describe the outcomes of urgency and urge incontinence after obliterative procedures or make any attempt to differentiate stress from urge incontinence. The authors of this text believe that, at a minimum, appropriate preoperative testing should be conducted to determine a postvoid residual urine and filling of the bladder with reduction maneuvers to demonstrate any potential occult or stress incontinence. If the patient has no significant postvoid residual volume and obvious occult or outright stress incontinence, then a synthetic sling could be considered concomitantly. If the patient has normal postvoid

Table 10-1 Collection of Literature on Obliterative Procedures

Citation	Study Summary	Recurrence	Malignancy	*De novo* Stress Urinary Incontinence	Conclusion
Hanson, 1969	Case series of 288 patients over 30 years showing >90% satisfaction	5 out of 288	1 out of 288	More urinary complaints such as *de novo* SUI as a result of distal dissections to the bladder neck	Le Fort colpocleisis is a safe and effective alternative for patients who do not require coital function.
Ubachs, 1973	Case series of 141 patients over 10 years 93 with follow-up examinations 84 of 93 patients satisfied with procedure	5 out of 93	0 out of 93	3 out of 93 with *de novo* SUI 15 out of 93 with some SUI including recurrence	Overall success rate is high with low postoperative morbidity. Rare cases of *de novo* SUI and recurrent prolapse are reported.
Moore, 2003	30 patients undergoing obliterative procedures with TVT; follow-up at 19 months	10% recurrent POP	No comment	6% recurrent or *de novo* SUI	Obliterative procedures performed with local anesthesia and sedation lead to high success and low morbidity.
Fitzgerald, 2003	Case series of 64 women undergoing colpocleisis; 33 with some antiincontinence procedures	3% recurrence	No comment	8 out of 64 with de *novo* SUI 3 out of 21 recurrent SUI after midurethral sling	High success rates for the treatment of prolapse symptoms achieved, but complicated decision making for incontinence management preoperatively and postoperatively.
von Pechmann et al, 2003	Case series of 92 patients undergoing colpocleisis over 12-year period Objective cure and subjective telephone interviews performed	56 out of 62 satisfied with results 97.8% objective cure rate (prolapse above the hymen)	0 out of 62	50% preoperative SUI 13% recurrent SUI postoperatively 90 out of 92 patients had some form of bladder neck suspension or sling	High success and satisfaction rates are reported with some recurrent and *de novo* SUIs.
Wheeler et al, 2005	Subjective success of partial colpocleisis in 32 patients using IIQ, UDI, and global satisfaction questionnaire Only 59% participation	Two patients	No comment	Improved UDI and IIQ scores	3 out of 32 (9%) regretted the procedure. 14% overall were not satisfied.
Hullfish, 2007	Subjective success of 93 patients undergoing colpocleisis Measured by IIQ, UDI, goal attainment	2.75 years follow-up with 95%-100% subjective relief of prolapse symptoms		Improvements in IIQ and UDI 84% stated goals met for urinary incontinence 2 out of 93 documented with *de novo* SUI	Low proportion of regret and high satisfaction with outcomes were reported after colpocleisis.
Fitzgerald et al, 2008	Pelvic Floor Disorders Network multicenter study of 152 patients with stages III to IV POP undergoing colpocleisis Evaluated by subjective measures including PFDI and PFIQ	95% satisfaction rate with 73% objective success of 92% for stages I-II	1 out of 152 patients with endometrial cancer 1 out of 152 with bladder cancer	47% underwent antiincontinence procedures 13% *de novo* SUI 14% recurrent incontinence	Overall favorable anatomic success at 1 year. SUI rates were consistent with previous reports. 94% of patients were satisfied; low rates of dissatisfaction by body image scale. Higher total blood loss with partial colpocleisis versus total colpocleisis.

Table 10-1 Collection of Literature on Obliterative Procedures—cont'd

Citation	Study Summary	Recurrence	Malignancy	De novo Stress Urinary Incontinence	Conclusion
Brubaker, 2009	Case series of 37 women undergoing colpocleisis and concomitant midurethral sling 30% with elevated PVR volume preoperatively Postoperative evaluation of urinary retention 3-month follow-up examination and telephone interview	Three patients had small rectocele at 3 months postoperatively	No comment	17 out of 37 had preoperative incontinence 11 persisted after midurethral sling 5 de novo SUI noted on telephone interview 2 out of 37 with elevated PVR volume	Concomitant midurethral sling may be placed in patients with colpocleisis even if preoperative PVR volume is elevated. Satisfaction rates were overall high.
Abbasy, 2010	Literature review of obliterative procedures Success rates, 90%-100% Postoperative regrets, 0%-12.9%	Low recurrence rates	No comment	Literature does not clearly define need for concomitant midurethral sling	High success rates and low proportion of regret were reported. Some de novo urinary symptoms developed but overall morbidity rates were low.

IIQ, Incontinence Impact Questionnaire; PFDI, Pelvic Floor Distress Inventory; PFIQ, Pelvic Floor Impact Questionnaire; POP, pelvic organ prolapse; PVR, elevated postvoid residual; SUI, stress urinary incontinence; TVT, tension-free vaginal tape; UDI, Urogenital Distress Inventory.

residual volume and no occult incontinence, then the authors recommend, at minimum, a Kelley-Kennedy plication of the bladder neck to prevent *de novo* stress incontinence. Alternatively, if a high postvoid residual volume is identified preoperatively, regardless of the outcome of the filling study or the presence of stress incontinence symptoms, the authors prefer not to perform any antiincontinence or suburethral plication with the concern of worsening voiding dysfunction. Postoperative stress incontinence can be then handled with a return to the surgical department for a midurethral sling or the injection of a bulk enhancing agent. Table 10-1 reviews the outcomes of the published literature on obliterative procedures.

SUMMARY: Obliterative procedures for advanced pelvic organ prolapse are increasing as a result of a growing number of aging older women in whom medical issues make more extensive surgery less suitable. Optimal treatment is contingent on a thorough assessment of historic and physical examination findings and an understanding of the relationship of the advanced prolapse and any co-existing visceral abnormalities. Obliterative surgeries have a very high rate of cure and satisfaction, and most of the morbidity is the result of preexisting medical conditions.

Suggested Readings

Abbasy S, Lowenstein L, Pham T, et al: Urinary retention is uncommon after colpocleisis with concomitant mid-urethral sling, *Int Urogynecol J Pelvic Floor Dysfunct* 20(2):213–216, 2009.

Abbasy S, Kenton K: Obliterative procedures for pelvic organ prolapse, *Clin Obstet Gynecol* 53(1):86–98, 2010.

Agarwala N, Hasiak N, Shade M: Graft interposition colpocleisis, perineorrhaphy, and tension-free sling for pelvic organ prolapse and stress urinary incontinence in elderly patients, *J Minim Invasive Gynecol* 14(6):740–745, 2007.

Barber MD, Amundsen CL, Paraiso MFR, et al: Quality of life after surgery for genital prolapse in elderly women: obliterative and reconstructive surgery, *Int Urogynecol J* 18:799–806, 2007.

Denehy TR, Choe JY, Gregori CA, et al: Modified Le Fort partial colpocleisis with Kelly urethral plication and posterior colpoperineoplasty in the medically compromised elderly: a comparison with vaginal hysterectomy, anterior colporrhaphy, and posterior colpoperineoplasty, *Am J Obstet Gynecol* 173:1697–1701, 1995.

DeLancey JO, Morley GW. Total colpocleisis for vaginal eversion, *Am J Obstet Gynecol* 176:1228-1232; discussion 1232-1235, 1997.

Fitzgerald MP, Brubaker L: Colpocleisis and urinary incontinence, *Am J Obstet Gynecol* 189:1241-1244, 2003.

Fitzgerald MP, Richter HE, Bradley CS, et al: Pelvic support, pelvic symptoms, and patient satisfaction after colpocleisis, *Int Urogynecol J Pelvic Floor Dysfunct* 19(2):1603-1609, 2008.

Gerten KA, Markland AD, Lloyd LK, et al: Prolapse and incontinence surgery in older women, *J Urol* 179(6):2111-2118, 2008.

Goldman J, Ovadia J, Feldberg D: The Neugebauer-Le Fort operation: a review of 118 partial colpo-cleises, *Eur J Obstet Gynecol Reprod Biol* 12:31-35, 1981.

Hanson GE, Keettel WC: The Neugebauer-Le Fort operation. A review of 288 colpocleises, *Obstet Gyne-cology* 34(3):352-357, 1969

Harmanli OH, Dandolu V, Chatwani AJ, et al: Total colpocleisis for severe pelvic organ prolapse, *J Reprod Med* 48:703-706, 2003.

Hullfish KL, Bovbjerg VE, Steers WD: Colpocleisis for pelvic organ prolapse: patient goals, quality of life, and satisfaction, *Obstet Gynecol* 110(2 Pt 1):341-345, 2007.

Linda Brubaker Urinary retention is uncommon after colpocleisis with concomitant mid-urethral sling, *Int Urogynecol J* 20:213-216, 2009.

Moore RD, Miklos JR: Colpocleisis and tension-free vaginal tape sling for severe uterine and vaginal prolapse and stress urinary incontinence under local anesthesia, *J Am Assoc Gynecol Laparosc* 10(2):276-280, 2003.

Stepp KJ, Barber MD, Eun-Hee Y, et al: Incidence of perioperative complications of urogynecologic surgery in elderly women, *Am J Obstet Gynecol* 192:1630-1636, 2005.

Ubachs JM, van Sante TJ, Schellekens LA: Partial colpocleisis by a modification of Le Fort's operation, *Obstet Gynecol* 42(3):415-420, 1973.

von Pechmann WS, Mutone M, Fyffe J, et al: Total Colpocleisis with high levator plication for the treatment of advanced pelvic organ prolapse, *Am J Obstet Gynecol* 189(1):121-126, 2003.

Walter S, von Pechmann MD, Martina Mutone MD, et al: Total colpocleisis with high levator plication for the treatment of advanced pelvic organ prolapse, *Am J Obstet Gynecol* 189:121-126, 2003.

Wheeler TL 2nd, Richter HE, Burgio KL, et al: Regret, satisfaction, and symptom improvement: analysis of the impact of partial colpocleisis for the management of severe pelvic organ prolapse, *Am J Obstet Gynecol* 193(6):2067-2070, 2005.

Surgery for Pelvic Organ Prolapse: Avoiding and Managing Complications

11

Mickey Karram MD and Christopher F. Maher MD

 Video Clips online

11-1 Intraoperative Management of Ureteral Kink during Vaginal Repair of Prolapse
11-2 Postoperative Management of Ureteral Obstruction after Vaginal Prolapse Repair
11-3 Vaginal Repair of Cystotomy
11-4 Laparoscopic View of Cystotomy and Ureteral Injury after Laparoscopic-Assisted Vaginal Hysterectomy
11-5 Recurrent Prolapse with Mesh Erosion after Trocar-Based Vaginal Mesh Kit
11-6 Vaginal Mesh Erosion Managed with Surgisis Biodesign
11-7 Recurrent Vaginal Mesh Erosion Managed with Surgisis Biodesign
11-8 Excision of Synthetic Mesh from the Rectum
11-9 Laparoscopic Evaluation and Management of Postoperative Bowel Dysfunction

11-10 Vaginal Repair of Vesicovaginal Fistula with Removal of Biologic Graft from the Wall of the Bladder
11-11 Techniques of How to Take Down Distal Iatrogenic Vaginal Constriction
11-12 Technique of How to Take Down Constriction with the Use of a Postoperative Vaginal Mold
11-13 Vaginal Excision of Mesh Causing Postoperative Vaginal Pain and Dyspareunia
11-14 Laparoscopic Excision of Mesh from the Bladder
11-15 Vaginal Removal of Mesh from the Bladder

This chapter reviews a variety of potential complications that can occur during or as a result of surgical repair for pelvic organ prolapse. All cases and discussions have one or more accompanying video clips that demonstrate the technical aspects of managing the various complications.

Case 1: Intraoperative Management of Ureteral Kink during a Vaginal Prolapse Repair

 View: Videos 11-1 and 11-2

A 56-year-old patient with symptomatic pelvic organ prolapse undergoes a vaginal prolapse repair, which involves an anterior colporrhaphy and a vaginal vault suspension to the uterosacral ligaments. After completing the anterior colporrhaphy and tying of the apical stitches to suspend the vaginal vault, 5 ml intravenous indigo carmine is administered and a cystourethroscopy is performed to ensure ureteral patency. Prompt efflux of dye is observed from the right ureter;

however, no efflux is observed from the left ureter 15 minutes after administering the dye. Close visualization of the ureter reveals peristalsis of the intravesical part of the ureter.

Case Discussion

This example of a ureteral kink or obstruction is typical of one that has occurred secondary to a prolapse repair. Either the stitches placed through the uterosacral ligament on the patient's left side or one of the stitches placed for the anterior colporrhaphy has caused the obstruction. Options to address this obstruction could involve attempting to pass a stent or performing a retrograde study. However, in the author's opinion, the next step of management should be to identify the suture causing the obstruction, cut it, ensure ureteral patency, and then, if appropriate, replace the suture. In this particular case, the offending suture is from the anterior colporrhaphy; once the suture is cut, immediate visualization of dye is noted. The suture is replaced, and ureteral patency is again ensured; the procedure is completed. (**See Video 11-1, "Intraoperative Management of Ureteral Kink during Vaginal Repair of Prolapse," and Video 11-2, "Postoperative Management of Ureteral Obstruction after Vaginal Prolapse Repair,"** for demonstrations of how best to address a ureteral kink during and after a vaginal prolapse repair.)

Case 2: Management of Inadvertent Cystotomy during Vaginal Prolapse Repair

 View: Video 11-3

A 65-year-old woman has recurrent vaginal prolapse, mostly secondary to a large cystocele. The patient has consented for a mesh-augmented repair of her recurrent cystocele. During the anterior vaginal wall dissection of the bladder off the vaginal wall, an inadvertent cystotomy occurs. (**See Video 11-3, "Vaginal Repair of Cystotomy."**) The dissection proceeds, and the cystotomy is completely mobilized off the vaginal wall to allow a tension-free closure. A vaginal sponge or packing is placed in the vagina to maintain a relatively watertight seal, and the cystoscopy is undertaken to view the ureteral orifices and to determine the distance from the cystotomy to the ureters to ensure that a safe closure can be accomplished without compromising either ureter. If the cystotomy is in close proximity to one or both ureteral orifices, then the authors recommend the placement of ureteral catheters during the repair of the cystotomy. The catheters may have to be maintained in place if postoperative edema or swelling is a concern. The cystotomy is then closed in layers with a fine delayed absorbable suture. The authors recommend either 3-0 Vicryl or chromic sutures. The authors prefer to interrupt the first layer, which should involve a mucosa-to-mucosa closure with a second layer imbricating the muscularis over the first layer. The mesh augmentation portion of the procedure is abandoned as a result of the concerns about the mesh being in contact with the cystotomy, which could create a potential infection, the breakdown of the cystotomy, or an erosion of the mesh into the bladder. The authors recommend proceeding with a vaginal suture repair of the cystocele to correct the anterior vaginal wall prolapse. The remainder of the repairs is performed as initially planned. The bladder is continuously drained with an indwelling Foley catheter for 10 to 14 days, depending on the size and location of the defect. A cystogram that confirms an intact bladder is recommended before removing the catheter. A voiding cystogram also ensures that the patient is able to void spontaneously in an efficient fashion when the catheter is removed.

Case 3: Laparoscopic View of Cystotomy and Ureteral Injury after Laparoscopic-Assisted Vaginal Hysterectomy

 View: Video 11-4

A 46-year-old woman with mildly symptomatic uterovaginal prolapse and some uterine fibroids undergoes a laparoscopic-assisted vaginal hysterectomy. A urogynecologic consultation is obtained to address a large cystotomy that occurred during the laparoscopic dissection of the bladder off the lower uterine segment. During the laparoscopic assessment of the cystotomy, a large defect is noted; in addition, no efflux of urine or dye is observed spilling from the right ureteral orifice. An attempt at passing a ureteral catheter is unsuccessful. After administering intravenous indigo carmine, intraperitoneal dye confirms a right ureteral injury. **(See Video 11-4, "Laparoscopic View of Cystotomy and Ureteral Injury after Laparoscopic-Assisted Vaginal Hysterectomy."**) Urologic consultation is obtained to perform a ureteral reimplantation procedure.

Discussion of Cases 2 and 3

These two cases depict how best to manage intraoperative injuries to the lower urinary tract that can occur during pelvic reconstructive surgery. Identifying and addressing any injury intraoperatively whenever possible are extremely important. Although an injury might be noted only in the bladder, one should not assume that an injury to one or both ureters has not also occurred. A full assessment of ureteral patency and bladder integrity should be undertaken whenever any concern exists that the lower urinary tract might have been compromised during pelvic reconstructive surgery.

Case 4: Vaginal Mesh Erosion after Total Vaginal Mesh Kit with Trocar-Based System

 View: Videos 11-5, 11-6, 11-7

A 59-year-old woman has recurrent pelvic organ prolapse and erosion of a large piece of mesh into the upper part of the anterior vaginal wall. She underwent a trocar-based total vaginal mesh kit repair 6 months before presentation. Her symptoms now include a feeling of recurrent prolapse, significant dyspareunia related to the mesh erosion, and vaginal bleeding and discharge. An examination reveals apical prolapse with descent of Point C to −1, as well as recurrent prolapse of the upper part of the anterior vaginal wall (Point Ba at 0). A vaginal excision of the eroded mesh is performed with a suture repair of her apical prolapse and recurrent cystocele. **(See Video 11-5, "Recurrent Prolapse with Mesh Erosion after Trocar-Based Vaginal Mesh Kit."**)

Case Discussion

This erosion most likely occurred as a result of a bunching up of the mesh in the anterior vaginal wall. Failure of a prolapse repair after a mesh kit does not exclude a patient from a subsequent native-tissue suture repair. During dissection of the anterior vaginal wall, the peritoneum was entered, and a high uterosacral vaginal vault suspension was accomplished to suspend the prolapsed cuff adequately. The mesh was sharply excised, and the recurrent cystocele was corrected with an anterior colporrhaphy. Mesh erosions after prolapse repair can be quite challenging, especially if they are large and occur high in the vagina. Any underlying infection should be treated preoperatively, followed by 2 weeks of oral antibiotics. If the vaginal mucosa cannot be closed without tension, a Surgisis Biodesign biologic graft (Cook Medical) can be sutured into the defect; it will convert to vaginal epithelium with healing. **(See Videos 11-5, "Recurrent Prolapse with Mesh Erosion after Trocar-Based Vaginal Mesh Kit"; Video 11-6, "Vaginal Mesh Erosion Managed with Surgisis Biodesign"; and Video 11-7, "Recurrent Vaginal Mesh Erosion Managed with Surgisis Biodesign"** for examples of how best to manage vaginal mesh erosions.)

Case 5: Rectal Injury as a Result of a Trocar-Based Posterior Vaginal Mesh Kit

 View: Videos 11-8, 11-9

A 62-year-old woman has a history of having a trocar-based mesh kit placed in a posterior vaginal wall approximately 18 months before presentation. Since the placement of this mesh, she has experienced significant vaginal pain, as well as recurrent infections with intermittent foul-smelling discharge from the pararectal incisions occurring approximately every 6 weeks. A rectal examination reveals one of the arms of the mesh kit has clearly transected the lumen of the rectum. A rectovaginal fistula with mesh eroding into the posterior vaginal wall is also noted. After a colorectal consultation and a detailed discussion with the patient, the decision is made to proceed with an attempt at vaginal excision of the mesh without diverting her bowel. Intravenous antibiotics are administered, and full-bowel preparation is performed before the surgery. At the time of the examination, the tissue was not believed to be extremely indurated; and clinically, no ongoing active infection was evident; these facts were the basis for the decision to proceed without diversion. The patient fully understood the possibility of a breakdown of the repair and the subsequent necessity to have diversion if the attempt of mesh removal proved unsuccessful. The mesh is successfully removed from the vagina and rectum, and the rectovaginal fistula is repaired. **(See Video 11-8, "Excision of Synthetic Mesh from the Rectum."** **)** The patient healed with no breakdown of any portion of the surgery.

Case Discussion

This case clearly depicts a technical failure on the part of the surgeon who placed the mesh kit. An adequate rectal examination at the time of surgery should have been performed, which would have allowed the surgeon to determine that the rectum was perforated with the mesh arm. In such a situation, the mesh that had transected the rectum should have been removed and the entire procedure aborted to allow proper healing of the rectal injury. If an enterotomy were to occur at the time of the laparoscopic surgery or open sacral colpopexy, then the defect should be repaired and the colpopexy with synthetic mesh placement should be abandoned in the opinion of the authors. Patients with bowel symptoms (especially obstruction) that date back to a surgical intervention should be considered for laparoscopic evaluation, assuming all other investigations are negative. **Video 11-9, "Laparoscopic Evaluation and Management of Postoperative Bowel Dysfunction,"** demonstrates some cases of pathologic abnormalities that can be identified at the time of laparoscopy in patients with postoperative bowel symptoms after repair of pelvic organ prolapse.

Case 6: Vesicovaginal Fistula after Cystocele Augmented with Biologic Graft

View: Video 11-10

A 76-year-old patient has an obvious vesicovaginal fistula arising from the midportion of the anterior vaginal wall. A cystocele repair, augmented with a biologic material (Pelvicol), was performed approximately 6 months before presentation. Cystoscopic examination reveals the fistula to be in the midtrigone well below the ureteral orifices; however, obvious bunching up of the Pelvicol is observed just under the mucosa of the bladder extending in close proximity to the right ureteral orifice. The plan is to place bilateral double-J stents and proceed with a vaginal repair of the vesicovaginal fistula with excision of the Pelvicol from the wall of the bladder. The procedure is accomplished without incident, and the patient has successful closure of the fistula after 2 weeks of continuous postoperative drainage. **(See Video 11-10, "Vaginal Repair of Vesicovaginal Fistula with Removal of Biologic Graft from the Wall of the Bladder."** **)**

Case Discussion

An undiagnosed bladder injury occurred at the time of the initial repair as a result of the fact that the surgeon was in a dissection plane that was most likely in the wall of the bladder. This case depicts the importance of fully mobilizing the vaginal wall in an appropriate plane off the bladder before cystocele repair, with or without any augmentation material.

Case 7: Vaginal Pain and Dyspareunia after Native Tissue Prolapse Repair

 View: Videos 11-11, 11-12

After a vaginal hysterectomy and anterior and posterior colporrhaphy performed 6 months earlier, a 45-year-old patient has primary complaints of the inability to have intercourse, secondary to her partner not being able to penetrate her vagina. Approximately 2.5 cm inside the introitus, an examination reveals a vaginal constriction ring that is fairly tight and sensitive. The examiner is only able to pass one finger through the constriction ring. The vaginal length appears to be adequate, and the vagina above the constriction seems fairly normal. The plan is to proceed with a takedown of the constriction ring by making bilateral relaxing incisions through the constriction band using a monopolar cautery device and then allowing the vagina to heal by secondary intention. **(See Video 11-11, "Techniques of How to Take Down Distal Iatrogenic Vaginal Constriction."**).

Case Discussion

This case depicts a situation in which too much vaginal wall was most likely trimmed during the anterior and posterior colporrhaphy, resulting in some scarring and constriction of the vaginal wall. Other possibilities are that the patient was not examined during the postoperative period and some inappropriate scarification developed that could have been prevented by early intervention with examinations and the possible use of a vaginal dilator. The two videos demonstrating how to address postoperative vaginal constriction both use monopolar cautery to release the vaginal constriction completely. A self-styled mold can be inserted into the vagina to minimize the risk of reformation of a vaginal constriction or the patient must undergo frequent postoperative examinations. Either way, the vagina will heal by secondary intention and vaginal dilators are regularly used until regular coital activity is feasible. If a mold is used, then it is sutured in place with vulvar sutures with an indwelling Foley catheter in place for approximately 2 weeks. The patient is maintained on oral antibiotics. **(See Video 11-11, "Techniques of How to Take Down Distal Iatrogenic Vaginal Constriction," and Video 11-12, "Technique of How to Take Down Constriction with the Use of a Postoperative Vaginal Mold."**)

Case 8: Vaginal Mesh Kit Causing Significant Vaginal Pain and Dyspareunia

 View: Video 11-13

A 56-year-old patient has significant vaginal pain after previous trocar-based mesh kit repair. No obvious erosion of the mesh is revealed on examination; however, in the upper part of the anterior and posterior vaginal wall, the mesh is easily palpated underneath a thin tight vaginal wall that is extremely tender. The plan is to remove the mesh from these tender areas to release the tension from the arms of the mesh and thus reduce the patient's pain. On opening the vaginal wall over the tender areas, the mesh is noted to be thick and under significant tension. The mesh is sharply excised and the vagina closed. Although the patient has noted a reduction in her pain, she continues to have intermittent vaginal pain and some dyspareunia. **(See Video 11-13, "Vaginal Excision of Mesh Causing Postoperative Vaginal Pain and Dyspareunia."**)

Case Discussion

When this situation occurs, the trocar arms of the mesh kit were most likely inappropriately passed, which resulted in shrinkage and bunching up of the mesh. Great care must be taken to appropriately trim and lay the mesh flat and to ensure that the arms are not under tension. Anteriorly, the arms need to be separated appropriately from each other and passed through the obturator membrane near the origin and insertion of the arcus tendineus fascia pelvis. If the two arms of an anterior mesh kit are passed in close proximity to each other, then bunching up of the mesh will ultimately result, which can be a precursor to excessive shrinking and vaginal pain.

Women who develop mesh contraction after surgery will subsequently experience vaginal and suprapubic pain, which is worse with coitus, movement, and sitting. An examination usually reveals a vagina that is well supported, and palpation identifies localized area of tight contracted mesh under the vaginal mucosa. Palpation of the localized area of mesh contraction reproduces the pain the patient experiences. Mesh erosions will occur in up to 50% of these patients. The pain in these patients can be debilitating. The surgical treatment of this condition involves the removal of the contracted portion of the mesh. The surgery is usually performed vaginally but can also be performed laparoscopically if the upper portion of the mesh is tight and contracted. **(See Video 13, "Vaginal Excision of Mesh Causing Postoperative Vaginal Pain and Dyspareunia."**)

Principles of excision of contracted mesh include identifying the contracted tight mesh under the vaginal mucosa, mobilizing the vagina from the tight mesh, mobilizing the bladder or bowel from the mesh, and removing as large a segment of tight mesh as feasible to ensure the body of the mesh is detached from the arms. The surgeon must be prepared to deal with any potential injury to the bowel or urinary tract.

Case 9: Surgical Excision of Intravesical Mesh after Trocar-Based Anterior Vaginal Prolapse

 View: Videos 11-14, 11-15

A 52-year-old woman is referred after cystoscopic examination, which revealed intravesical mesh. She had undergone a total vaginal mesh repair for prolapse 2 years earlier. Her presenting symptoms are recurrent urinary tract infections and constant irritative symptoms in the form of urinary urgency and frequency.

The following two techniques are demonstrated to remove mesh from the bladder.

Surgical Steps: Laparoscopic Excision of Mesh via a Transvesical Approach

This technique involves using the laparoscopic via a transvesical approach to the intravesical mesh. The improved vision and precision afforded with the transvesical approach facilitate the excision of any foreign body from the wall of the bladder.

1. A camera and three additional surgical 5-mm trocars are used.
2. A vertical incision with diathermy opens the bladder dome creating a high extraperitoneal cystotomy approximately 5 cm in length.
3. Intraabdominal gas quickly distends the bladder and affords excellent visualization.
4. The mesh invariably breaches the mucosa in the trigone, and ureteric catheters are introduced via the urethra; the ureters are cannulated bilaterally.
5. With traction on the mesh, the mesh is mobilized from the bladder mucosa using sharp dissection.
6. The mesh is then mobilized from the vagina and excised at the point where the mesh is incorporated in tissue.
7. The bladder mucosa is mobilized from the vagina.
8. A precise and careful single-layer closure without tension is performed on the bladder mucosa.
9. Ureteric catheters are removed, and patency is confirmed.
10. Routine closure of the dome incision is performed in two layers with continuous 2.0 Vicryl sutures.
11. The indwelling Foley catheter is inserted into the bladder and left for 10 days; a cystogram confirms no extravasation of contrast medium before the catheter is removed. **(See Video 11-14, "Laparoscopic Excision of Mesh from the Bladder."**)

Surgical Steps: Transvaginal Excision of Mesh from the Bladder

The second of the two techniques involves a transvaginal approach to remove mesh from the bladder.

1. Bilateral double-J ureteral stents are placed.

2. The vaginal mucosa is opened, and the vaginal epithelium is dissected off the underlying mesh.

3. The full thickness of the mesh is incised at a point where the mesh is not in the bladder.

4. Sharp dissection is used to mobilize the mesh off the wall of the bladder.

5. All intravesical mesh is sharply excised from the bladder.

6. The cystotomy is closed without tension in two layers.

7. The vaginal epithelium is closed.

   See Video 11-15, "Vaginal Removal of Mesh from the Bladder."

Index

Page numbers followed by "f" indicate
figures, "t" indicate tables, and "b"
indicate boxes.

Printed and bound by CPI Group (UK) Ltd, Croydon, CR0 4YY

08/05/2025

01864793-0002